AF802637

Trust Carol J. Buck and Elsevier
to take you through the levels of coding success

Step 4: Professional Resources

Step 3: Certify

Step 2: Practice

Step 1: Learn

With the resources you need for every level of coding success, Carol J. Buck and Elsevier are with you every step of your coding career. From beginning to advanced, from the classroom to the workplace, from application to certification, the Step Series products are your guides to greater opportunities and successful career advancement.

Keep climbing with the most trusted name in medical coding.

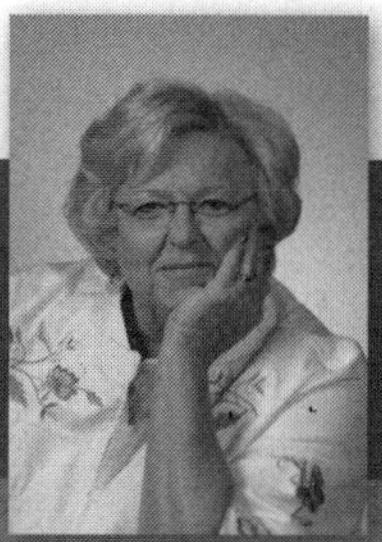

Author and Educator
Carol J. Buck, MS, CPC, CPC-H, CCS-P

-00

Step 3: Certify

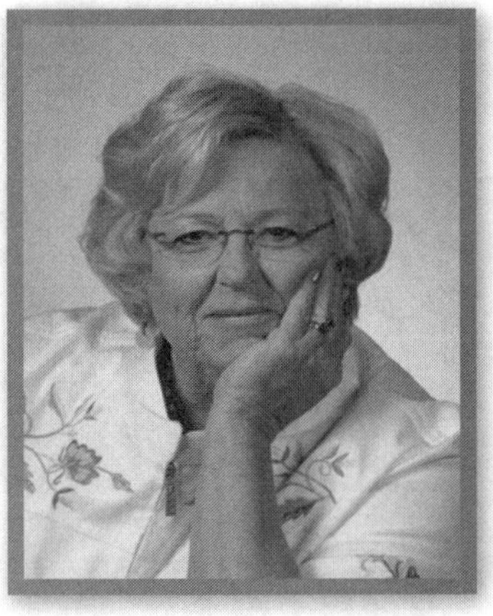

Congratulations on reaching the certification step in your career! As you know, certified coders are in top demand in today's marketplace. That's why, as a lifelong coder and educator, I have dedicated myself to providing the most up-to-date, comprehensive, and user-friendly certification review books on the market. I update this book every year so that you will have the best tool possible when studying for your certification exam. It's time to hit the books. ***You can do it! I know you can!***

— Carol J. Buck, MS, CPC, CPC-H, CCS-P

Track your progress!

See the checklist in the back of this book to learn more about your next step toward coding success!

2012 THE PRACTICE STEP

Physician-Based Coding Cases

2012 THE PRACTICE STEP

Physician-Based Coding Cases

CAROL J. BUCK, MS, CPC, CPC-H, CCS-P
Former Program Director
Medical Secretary Programs
Northwest Technical College
East Grand Forks, Minnesota

ELSEVIER

ELSEVIER
SAUNDERS

3251 Riverport Lane
St. Louis, Missouri 63043

THE PRACTICE STEP: PHYSICIAN-BASED CODING CASES

ISBN: 978-1-4557-0753-9

Notices

Knowledge and best practice in this field are constantly changing. As new research and experience broaden our understanding, changes in research methods, professional practices, or medical treatment may become necessary.

Practitioners and researchers must always rely on their own experience and knowledge in evaluating and using any information, methods, compounds, or experiments described herein. In using such information or methods they should be mindful of their own safety and the safety of others, including parties for whom they have a professional responsibility.

With respect to any drug or pharmaceutical products identified, readers are advised to check the most current information provided (i) on procedures featured or (ii) by the manufacturer of each product to be administered, to verify the recommended dose or formula, the method and duration of administration, and contraindications. It is the responsibility of practitioners, relying on their own experience and knowledge of their patients, to make diagnoses, to determine dosages and the best treatment for each individual patient, and to take all appropriate safety precautions.

To the fullest extent of the law, neither the Publisher nor the authors, contributors, or editors, assume any liability for any injury and/or damage to persons or property as a matter of products liability, negligence or otherwise, or from any use or operation of any methods, products, instructions, or ideas contained in the material herein.

NOTE: *Current Procedural Terminology, 2012,* was used in updating this text.

Library of Congress Cataloging-in-Publication Data

Buck, Carol J.
The practice step : physician-based coding cases / Carol J. Buck. -- 2012 ed.
p. ; cm.
Rev. ed. of: The extra step / Carol J. Buck, Jacqueline Klitz Grass. 2011.
ISBN 978-1-4557-0753-9 (pbk. :alk. paper) 1. Nosology--Code numbers--Problems, exercises, etc. I. Buck, Carol J. Extra step. II. Title.
[DNLM: 1. Clinical Coding--Problems and Exercises. 2. Practice Management, Medical--Problems and Exercises. W 18.2]
RB115.B825 2011b
651.5′04261--dc23

2011028112

Publisher: Jeanne R. Olson
Developmental Editor: Diane Chatman
Publishing Services Manager: Pat Joiner-Myers
Project Manager: Marlene Weeks
Senior Designer: Amy Buxton

Printed in the United States of America

Last digit is the print number: 9 8 7 6 5 4 3 2 1

Development of This Edition

This book would not have been possible without a team of educators and professionals, including practicing coders and technical consultants. The combined efforts of the team members have made this text an incredible learning tool.

LEAD TECHNICAL COLLABORATOR

Jacqueline Klitz Grass, MA, CPC
Coding and Reimbursement Specialist
Altru Health System
Grand Forks, North Dakota

SENIOR CODING SPECIALIST

Lindsay-Anne Jenkins, CRNA, CPC, CPC-H, CPC-I, CIRCC, CANPC
Coding and Auditing Specialist
St. Louis, Missouri

SENIOR ICD-10-CM AND ICD-9-CM CODING SPECIALIST

Karla R. Lovaasen, RHIA, CCS, CCS-P
Coding and Consulting Services
Abingdon, Maryland

—Co-author of *2012 ICD-9-CM Coding: Theory and Practice with ICD-10,* St. Louis, 2012, Saunders.
—Co-author of *ICD-10-CM/PCS Coding: Theory and Practice, 2012 Edition,* St. Louis, 2012, Saunders.

SENIOR COLLABORATOR AND ICD-10-CM CONSULTANT

Nancy Maguire, ACS, CRT, PCS, FCS, HCS-D, APC, AFC
Physician Consultant for Auditing and Education
Universal City, Texas

QUERY MANAGER

Patricia Cordy Henricksen, MS, CHCA, CPC-I, CPC, CCP-P, PCS
Approved PMCC Instructor
Education Director, Lexington Local Chapter of AAPC
Bluegrass Medical Managers Association
Lexington, Kentucky

QUERY TEAM

Debra Kroll, RHIT
Denial and Billing Compliance Supervisor
Altru Health System
Grand Forks, North Dakota

Introduction

The skill of medical coding is acquired through many long hours of practice. It is not a skill that can be learned simply by reading about code assignment. Only through a detailed analysis of a wide variety of reports can the coder be proficient. Once you have coded a particular service or diagnosis, you have improved your knowledge base and you will find it is easier the next time you code that particular service or diagnosis. The key words to improve your coding ability are patience and practice.

This product can be used to assist you in improving your coding ability in a specific coding area or for experience in a broad array of specialty areas. Users have found these real-life reports are helpful in preparing for certification examinations, such as the CPC, because these reports provide experience in coding many physician services.

The text is composed of 18 chapters:

Chapter 1 Evaluation and Management
Chapter 2 Anesthesiology
Chapter 3 Cardiology
Chapter 4 Integumentary
Chapter 5 Emergency Medicine
Chapter 6 Medicine
Chapter 7 Gastroenterology
Chapter 8 Nephrology
Chapter 9 Neurology and Ophthalmology
Chapter 10 Obstetrics and Gynecology
Chapter 11 Orthopedics
Chapter 12 Otorhinolaryngology
Chapter 13 Pathology
Chapter 14 Pediatrics, Neonatology, and Adolescent Medicine
Chapter 15 Diagnostic Radiology
Chapter 16 Interventional Radiology and Radiation Oncology
Chapter 17 Urology
Chapter 18 General Surgery

There are a variable number of reports within each chapter to give you experience in each of these major coding areas. This edition features abstracting questions presented at the end of each report. These questions will assist you as you improve your critical thinking skills necessary to code medical reports. Your instructor has access to these answers via the Evolve website. Students not enrolled in a course do not have access to these answers.

Contents

CHAPTER 9: NEUROLOGY AND OPHTHALMOLOGY

CHAPTER 10: OBSTETRICS AND GYNECOLOGY

CHAPTER 11: ORTHOPEDICS

CHAPTER 15: DIAGNOSTIC RADIOLOGY

CHAPTER 16: INTERVENTIONAL RADIOLOGY AND RADIATION ONCOLOGY

CHAPTER 17: UROLOGY

Chapter 1

Evaluation and Management

Generally, facilities such as hospitals assign and report external cause/E codes. However, physician offices may choose to do so as well. The external cause/E code is to be assigned for the initial encounter, but not for subsequent encounters. For educational purposes, the external cause code is to be assigned when directed to do so throughout this manual. See ICD-10-CM Section I.C.20.a./ICD-9-CM Section I.C.19.a. of the Official Guidelines for Coding and Reporting for directions on external cause code/E code assignment.

Case 1-1: Discharge Summary, Chest Pain

DISCHARGE SUMMARY

LOCATION: Inpatient, Hospital

PATIENT: Jessy Stark

ATTENDING PHYSICIAN: George Orbitz, MD

Jessy is a 50-year-old Caucasian female who was admitted because of chest pain. She was found to have noncardiac chest pain. Her echocardiogram showed normal left ventricular function; no evidence of pericardial effusion; no evidence of pericarditis on physical exam or ECG. V/Q scan indicated noncardiac chest pain. She was reassured and was discharged in good general condition. Her code status is level I.

The patient will be followed up in my clinic within a week.

CPT Code(s): ______________________________

ICD-10-CM Code(s): ______________________________

ICD-9-CM Code(s): ______________________________

Abstracting Questions

1. Was the amount of time of the discharge service documented? ______________________________

(Answers to all Abstracting Questions are located on your Instructor's Evolve site. If you are not currently enrolled in a course, you will not have access to these answers. Record your responses to these questions and ask your instructor for the answers.)

Case 1-2: Progress Note, Acute and Chronic Renal Failure

PROGRESS NOTE

LOCATION: Inpatient, Hospital

PATIENT: Mike Lumbardi

ATTENDING PHYSICIAN: George Orbitz, MD

NEPHROLOGY PROGRESS NOTE: Mike had no major events. He tolerated the angiogram very well. He had peripheral vascular disease, but nothing to bypass, unfortunately. The patient denies any chest pain, shortness of breath. He has no nausea or vomiting. He has no leg edema and no GI symptoms.

PHYSICAL EXAMINATION: His vital signs were stable this morning. Temperature 36.9°C. Blood pressure 165/85. Heart rate 52 per minute. Respirations 16 per minute. Sats were 96% on room air. The patient was not in any respiratory, cardiac, or neurologic distress. He had no increase in jugulovenous pressure; regular rate and rhythm. The lungs were clear bilaterally without any crackles. The abdomen was soft and nontender; no organomegaly. No edema, with decreased pulses bilaterally, with signs of chronic venous and arterial insufficiency.

Intake/output in the past 8 hours: 1286 in, 1050 out.

Labs are pending from this morning, but his creatinine yesterday was 1.3.

IMPRESSION
1. Acute on top of chronic renal failure related to intravascular volume depletion, with creatinine coming down from 1.6 to 1.3.
2. Peripheral vascular disease.
3. Hypertension.

RECOMMENDATIONS
1. Basic metabolic panel is pending today.
2. If his creatinine goes up over time, he might need to have a renal MRA to look for renal artery stenosis.
3. Since patient is making urine, I don't think that his creatinine will go up acutely after his angiogram yesterday.

CPT Code(s): ____________________

ICD-10-CM Code(s): ____________________

ICD-9-CM Code(s): ____________________

Abstracting Questions

1. Are all three key elements (history, examination, and MDM complexity) documented? ____________
2. How many key elements are required for this type of service? ____________
3. Should both acute and chronic renal failure be reported, and if so, which is reported first? ____________
4. Is the volume depletion reported? ____________

Case 1-3: Progress Note, Hypotension

PROGRESS NOTE

LOCATION: Inpatient, Hospital

PATIENT: Fidel Marsh

ATTENDING PHYSICIAN: George Orbitz, MD

The patient is undergoing CAPD using 1.5%. He is feeling much better today after I gave him intravenous fluids overnight. He is happier and smiling and not dizzy anymore. Yesterday, on his CAPD, he had in one exchange 700 out and the other exchange he had −200. So far today he had 500-cc ultrafiltration.

The patient gets occasional chest pain. He has been doing that for the past few months. It is difficult to figure out whether this is cardiac or noncardiac. His troponins last night were negative.

All of his medications were held, including metoprolol, Imdur, clonidine, and minoxidil.

PHYSICAL EXAMINATION: On examination this morning he is not in any respiratory, cardiologic, or neurologic distress. No pallor, jaundice, or cyanosis. Blood pressure 140s/60s. Heart rate 75 per minute. Respirations 18 per minute. Saturations 96% on room air. Lungs are clear bilaterally without any crackles. He has regular rate and rhythm without any murmurs or pericardial friction rubs. Abdomen is soft and nontender. Extremities: No edema.

The patient is getting intravenous fluids at 150 cc/hour.

IMPRESSION
1. Orthostatic hypotension secondary to intravascular volume depletion and overmedicated with antihypertensives. It all seems to be getting better.
2. Chest pain occasionally, which could be angina.

PLAN
1. Decrease IV to 75 cc/hour.
2. Resume Imdur at 60 mg p.o. q.d.
3. Restart metoprolol at 50 mg p.o. b.i.d. instead of 150 mg b.i.d.
4. Encourage activity.
5. Give nitroglycerin p.r.n. for chest pain.
6. Continue current dialysis prescription with only 1.5% and see how he does overnight.
7. Target planned discharge Monday morning.

CPT Code(s): ______________________________

ICD-10-CM Code(s): ______________________________

ICD-9-CM Code(s): ______________________________

Abstracting Questions

1. In the interval history, is the chief complaint documented? ______________________________
2. What is CAPD? ______________________________
3. What is another name for orthostatic hypotension? ______________________________
4. What is orthostatic/postural hypotension? ______________________________

Case 1-4: Discharge Summary, Cardiac Catheterization

DISCHARGE SUMMARY

LOCATION: Inpatient, Hospital

PATIENT: Jane Stein

ATTENDING PHYSICIAN: George Orbitz, MD

REASON FOR HOSPITALIZATION: Cardiac catheterization with renal prophylaxis measures for underlying chronic renal failure.

SUMMARY OF HOSPITAL COURSE: Three days ago the patient was admitted and was rendered renal prophylaxis measures prior to a cardiac catheterization because of underlying chronic renal failure. She was given fenoldopam, Mucomyst, intravenous fluids, etc. Two days ago a cardiac catheterization was performed, which actually showed no significant lesions. There was also normal left ventricular function noted. The patient tolerated the procedure without any complications. The patient's renal function remained stable throughout this hospitalization to the time of discharge.

Labs at time of discharge: Sodium 136, potassium 3.8, chloride 104, CO_2 24.1, BUN and creatinine are 18/1.8, glucose 137, calcium 8.

INSTRUCTIONS TO THE PATIENT AND HER FAMILY

Activity Level: As tolerated.

Diet: Renal diabetic diet.

CURRENT MEDICATIONS
1. Enteric-coated aspirin 325 q.d.
2. Diltiazem CD 360 mg q.d.
3. Premarin 0.625 mg q.d.
4. Imdur 90 mg q.d.
5. Provera 2.5 mg q.d.
6. Toprol XL 50 mg q.d.
7. Unicap 1 cap q.d.
8. Paxil 20 mg q.d.
9. Zocor 10 mg q.d.
10. Cozaar 50 mg q.d.
11. Nitroglycerin 0.4-mg tabs sublingual p.r.n. chest pain.

FOLLOW-UP APPOINTMENT AND CARE
1. Follow-up with Dr. Green as directed.
2. Follow-up with Dr. Elhart of cardiology as directed.
3. Follow-up in my clinic in one week with a basic metabolic panel.

CONDITION ON DISCHARGE COMPARED WITH CONDITION ON ADMISSION: Stable.

DISCHARGE FINAL DIAGNOSES
1. Status post cardiac catheterization with no significant lesions identified. Please refer to Dr. Elhart's cardiac catheterization report.

2. Chronic renal failure (latest creatinine clearance is 53 ml/min with creatinine of 1.4, total volume of 1300 ml, and 120 mg of proteinuria performed on January 29), most likely secondary to the following:
   a. Hypertension.
   b. Type 2 diabetes mellitus.
   c. History of previous contrast nephropathy from previous cardiac catheterization/percutaneous transluminal coronary angioplasty/stent placement.
   d. Elderly age.
3. Degenerative joint disease.
4. Hyperlipidemia.
5. Depression.
6. Positive osteoporosis risk factors.

I have spent a total of 40 minutes discussing discharge plans with this patient.

CPT Code(s): ____________________

ICD-10-CM Code(s): ____________________

ICD-9-CM Code(s): ____________________

Abstracting Questions

1. Was the patient admitted and discharged on the same calendar date? ____________________
2. Is the patient in a global period from the previous cardiac catheterization? ____________________
3. Was the amount of time of the visit documented? ____________________

Case 1-5: Nephrology Consultation, Hypertension

NEPHROLOGY CONSULTATION

LOCATION: Outpatient, Clinic

PATIENT: Cynthia Naef

PRIMARY CARE PHYSICIAN: Ronald Green, MD

CONSULTANT: George Orbitz, MD

REASON FOR CONSULTATION: Uncontrolled hypertension.

Ms. Naef is a 50-year-old female I was asked to see by Dr. Green regarding uncontrolled hypertension.

The patient's blood pressure at home has been in the 160s–170s/100s–110s. She has no symptoms of elevated blood pressure, meaning no headaches, epistaxis, chest pain, tinnitus, or neurologic symptoms. She was just started on hydrochlorothiazide.

The patient was diagnosed with hypertension a year ago. She has been seeing Dr. Green for claudication and severe peripheral vascular disease. She had a cough from lisinopril, which was discontinued recently.

PAST MEDICAL HISTORY
1. Hypertension for a year.
2. Severe peripheral vascular disease and claudication.
3. No ischemic changes on the recent Cardiolite.
4. ACE inhibitor–induced cough.
5. Cholecystectomy.
6. Carpal tunnel surgery.
7. C-section.
8. Head surgery in 1975.
9. Appendectomy.

CURRENT MEDICATIONS
1. Propranolol 50 mg q.d.
2. Zocor 200 mg q.d.
3. Albuterol inhaler.
4. Baby aspirin 81 mg q.d.
5. Hydrochlorothiazide 25 mg q.d.

FAMILY HISTORY: She has one brother with hypertension. Father deceased age 50 of pancreatic cancer. Mother deceased age 40 of leukemia.

SOCIAL HISTORY: The patient is married. She is a housewife. She drinks four times a week. She has been trying to quit smoking, and she started on Zyban. She lives in Anytown.

GYNECOLOGIC HISTORY: She has been in menopause since age 38.

PHYSICAL EXAMINATION: The patient is not in any respiratory, cardiac, or neurologic distress. Weight 134 pounds. Temperature 97°F. Pulse 72 per minute. Blood pressure: Sitting 160/80 and standing 146/86. No apparent jaundice or cyanosis. No cervical lymphadenopathy.

Thyroid is not palpable. Lungs are clear bilaterally. Regular rate and rhythm. No renal bruits. Soft and nontender abdomen. No edema.

IMPRESSION: Uncontrolled hypertension. Could be related to renal artery stenosis, I suspect.

PLAN
1. Target blood pressure less than 130/85.
2. Obtain random aldosterone and renal levels.
3. Basic metabolic panel, magnesium, and urinalysis today.
4. Obtain a renal ultrasound.
5. Taper propranolol and start labetalol 300 mg p.o. b.i.d., and I gave her a prescription for that.
6. Keep hydrochlorothiazide.
7. Return to clinic in four weeks.
8. Discussed all the above with patient, and she seems to understand and agree with the plan.

Thank you for allowing me to advise you in the care of this patient.

CPT Code(s): ____________________

ICD-10-CM Code(s): ____________________

ICD-9-CM Code(s): ____________________

Abstracting Questions

1. Where is this service rendered? ____________________
2. Can a consultation be reported if the consultant orders further studies? ____________________
3. The patient has a return visit in 4 weeks. How would this return visit be reported? ____________________

Case 1-6: Nephrology Consultation, Chronic Renal Failure

NEPHROLOGY CONSULTATION

LOCATION: Outpatient, Clinic

PATIENT: Nate Jesse

PRIMARY CARE PHYSICIAN: Alma Naraquist, MD

CONSULTANT: George Orbitz, MD

REASON FOR CONSULTATION: Abnormal creatinine clearance and elevated creatinine.

The patient is a 69-year-old Caucasian male I was asked to see by Dr. Naraquist to render an opinion on the patient's abnormal creatinine clearance.

The patient had an elevated creatinine of 1.8 in July and 1.6 in January. His creatinine clearance in July was 47 ml/min, with a urine creatinine of 55.5 mg/dl and a 24-hour urine volume of 2675 ml. His hemoglobin was 11.1 with a hematocrit of 33.6 in July, with a sedimentation rate of 70 mm/hour. His 24-hour urine volume in May was 70 mg.

The patient had a CT scan in May that showed no hydronephrosis in the kidneys. His main complaint is feeling fatigued. He denies any chest pain or shortness of breath. He has no leg edema. The patient was told he had one functioning kidney.

PAST MEDICAL HISTORY
1. Hypertension for the past 2 years.
2. Coronary artery disease, status post two myocardial infarctions and two stents two years ago by Dr. Noonar.
3. History of thecal tumor in March of this year with thecal laminectomy with gross total resection.
4. History of diffuse large basal cell carcinoma.
5. Hypercholesterolemia.

CURRENT MEDICATIONS
1. Aspirin.
2. Centrum.
3. Endocet for pain.
4. Foltx.
5. Lopid 600 mg b.i.d.
6. Prinivil 20 mg b.i.d.
7. Procardia XL 60 mg q.d.
8. Tenormin 50 mg q.d.
9. Zocor 80 mg q.h.s.

ALLERGIES: No known drug allergies.

FAMILY HISTORY: The patient's sister had dialysis post valve surgery. His father deceased at 68. Mother deceased at 76 of a stroke. He has three brothers and two sisters.

SOCIAL HISTORY: The patient is a retired banker. His highest level of education was 10th grade. He has one daughter born in 1957. He drinks alcohol occasionally. He does not currently smoke. He used to smoke two packs a day for 30 years. The patient lives in Paradise Hills.

REVIEW OF SYSTEMS: General: Fatigue with no fever, chills, or night sweats. No change of weight or appetite. Respiratory: Negative. Cardiac: Negative. Gastrointestinal: Negative. Genitourinary: Negative. Skin: Negative. Musculoskeletal: Occasional arthritis and arthralgia, otherwise negative.

PHYSICAL EXAMINATION: Weight 207 pounds. Temperature 96°F. Pulse 72. Blood pressure: Sitting 116/58 and standing 120/70. The patient is not in any respiratory, cardiac, or neurologic distress. Slight pallor. No jaundice or cyanosis. No cervical adenopathy. Thyroid is not palpable. Lungs are clear bilaterally. A systolic murmur. Abdomen is soft and nontender. I cannot hear any renal bruits. No leg edema.

IMPRESSION
1. Chronic renal failure, probably related to either hypertensive nephrosclerosis or ischemic nephropathy with mild nephrotic range or proteinuria, less than a gram a day.
2. Anemia, which is probably related to chronic renal failure.

PLAN
1. Obtain a renal ultrasound.
2. We will obtain a basic metabolic panel, complete blood count, and iron studies today.
3. Based on the results of the studies, we might start him on erythropoietin and we might give him intravenous iron.
4. The patient has an appointment with Dr. Green.
5. The patient is claustrophobic, but we might have to consider doing renal MRA to look for renal arthrostenosis.
6. We will continue with same medications.
7. I have obtained spot urine protein/creatinine ratio so that we can follow that up.
8. The patient was advised not to take any nonsteroidal anti-inflammatory drugs.
9. He is to return to clinic in two weeks to review labs, ultrasounds, and further management.

CPT Code(s): ______________________________

ICD-10-CM Code(s): ______________________________

ICD-9-CM Code(s): ______________________________

Abstracting Questions

1. The patient has a return visit scheduled; can the physician still report a consultation? ______________
2. What was the reason for the consultation? ______________________________

Case 1-7: Discharge Summary, End-Stage Renal Disease

DISCHARGE SUMMARY

LOCATION: Inpatient, Hospital

PATIENT: Jim Bravo

ATTENDING PHYSICIAN: George Orbitz, MD

DISCHARGE DIAGNOSES
1. Questionable cellulitis.
2. Gouty arthritis.
3. Gangrenous toe.
4. End-stage renal disease, on chronic hemodialysis.
5. Diabetes.

HOSPITAL COURSE: The patient was admitted. He had some clinical evidence of cellulitis in his left upper extremity and around his elbow, but he was also noted to have tophi on his olecranon bursa. He was given IV antibiotics. He was noted to have redness and tenderness in his left big toe. It seemed to be gangrenous. Dr. Green was involved in his care. We thought that this could be cellulitis. He received Unasyn IV, but he continued to be debilitated and in pain. His uric acid has always been controlled, but he had gouty arthritis before, and he has chronic tophaceous gout evidenced by clinical examination. Finally, he was given steroids IV, which dramatically improved his pain, including the redness in his toe.

The patient tolerated hemodialysis well during the hospitalization. We did not change him to peritoneal dialysis.

DISCHARGE PLAN: The patient will be going home today. He will continue p.o. antibiotics. We will continue tapering doses of prednisone. We will start him with 60 mg q.d. and taper until off. We will schedule him to see Dr. Jayco to have discussions related to hemodialysis and peritoneal dialysis. Code level 1.

CPT Code(s): ______________________________

ICD-10-CM Code(s): ______________________________

ICD-9-CM Code(s): ______________________________

Abstracting Questions

1. What procedure did the patient have done while hospitalized? ______________________________
2. What specific manifestation of gout did the patient have? ______________________________

Case 1-8: Discharge Summary, Hydronephrosis

DISCHARGE SUMMARY

LOCATION: Inpatient, Hospital

PATIENT: Elida Gaddis

ATTENDING PHYSICIAN: Frank Gaul, MD

ADMITTING DIAGNOSES

Primary Diagnosis: Hydronephrosis.

Secondary Diagnoses
1. Hypertension.
2. Gastroesophageal reflux disease.
3. Anemia.
4. Leg pain.

DISCHARGE DIAGNOSES

Primary Diagnosis: Acute renal failure.

Secondary Diagnoses
1. Chronic renal failure.
2. Hypertension.
3. Gastroesophageal reflux disease.
4. Asthma.

HOSPITAL COURSE: Patient was admitted by Dr. Avila. Patient was taken to the operating suite. She underwent ureteral stent placement. There was concern that this might have been plugged. She underwent restenting. She continued to have problems with poor urinary output and renal functioning. She had consultations from nephrology, as well as by Dr. Smithson in Dr. Avila's absence. Patient ultimately ended up needing dialysis catheter placed and did undergo dialysis. She improved with her leg pain and stabilized her renal functioning. She did not have any complications during her hospitalization. She did have difficulty with ambulation. She did have assistance with physical therapy and did get consultation from the physiatrist.

LABORATORY RESULTS: Creatinine ranged from 5.1 to 1.5. Troponin was negative. Renal ultrasound did show marked hydronephrosis. This was repeated and continued to show the hydronephrosis. She had venous Doppler exams. She did not show any thrombophlebitis.

PROCEDURES
1. Cystoscopy with bilateral stent placement times two.
2. Placement of tunnel hemodialysis catheter and hemodialysis.

DISCHARGE PLAN: Patient was discharged to the nursing home for continued care. She will continue to be seen by nephrology for this, and Dr. Alanda will be her primary care physician.

CPT Code(s): ______________________________

ICD-10-CM Code(s): ______________________________

ICD-9-CM Code(s): ______________________________

Abstracting Questions

1. Dr. Avila, who also performed a surgical procedure, admitted this patient. Would Dr. Avila report the discharge? ______________________________
2. The attending is listed as Dr. Gaul. Was there a transfer of care and would that enable him to report the discharge? ______________________________

Case 1-9: Progress Note, Hemoptysis

PROGRESS NOTE

LOCATION: Inpatient, Hospital

PATIENT: Antonio Maciel

ATTENDING PHYSICIAN: George Orbitz, MD

The patient has been having more coughing, more shortness of breath. His cough seems to be wet, but he is not bringing up anything. He might have had some coughing with hemoptysis yesterday. His vital signs are stable. He is at least 500-cc positive balance.

He has acute jugular venous pressure on physical examination. Lungs have inspiratory and expiratory crackles. No edema. He is awake, alert, and oriented times three.

Oxygen saturation 93% on 3 liters.

IMPRESSION
1. Hemoptysis.
2. Hypoxic respiratory failure.

PLAN
1. I will try and do NG suction.
2. We will get a stat chest x-ray.
3. Will give him Atarax and will decide whether we will give him Bumex or not.

CPT Code(s): ____________________

ICD-10-CM Code(s): ____________________

ICD-9-CM Code(s): ____________________

Abstracting Questions

1. What is the category of E/M codes used to report this service? ____________________
2. Are all three key components documented? ____________________
3. Are all three key components required to report this service? ____________________

Case 1-10: Neurosurgery Consultation, Neck Injury

NEUROSURGERY CONSULTATION

Assign an external cause code/E code to indicate how the injury occurred.

LOCATION: Inpatient, Hospital

PATIENT: Mike Bahs

ATTENDING PHYSICIAN: Loren White, MD

CONSULTANT: Timothy Pleasant, MD

REASON FOR CONSULTATION: Rule out neck injury.

HISTORY: This patient is a 17-year-old male who was involved in a motor vehicle accident last night. He remembers driving down the road and the next thing he remembers was trying to reach for his cell phone at a stop sign after the accident. He does not remember any of the details. The car apparently went off the road and hit a tree. The patient is amnesiac for the event but does not believe he lost consciousness. His vehicle was apparently traveling 35-40 miles an hour. There was no report that he was ejected from the vehicle.

PAST MEDICAL HISTORY: He had childhood asthma.

MEDICATIONS: None.

ALLERGIES: None.

FAMILY HISTORY: Noncontributory to the present problem.

SOCIAL HISTORY: He chews tobacco. Alcohol use is rare.

EXAMINATION: Vital signs show he is afebrile. Pulse 64. Blood pressure 110/50. Neurologic: He is awake, alert, and fully oriented. His cranial nerves are grossly intact. HEENT: His extraocular movements are full. His eyes are conjugate. His pupils are equal. His facial strength is intact. On motor examination, he has grossly normal motor strength bilaterally in the upper and lower extremities. His reflexes are normal and symmetric at the biceps, triceps, and brachioradialis. The ankle jerks and the knee jerks are normal and symmetric. Gait is not tested. Sensory examination is grossly intact to light touch. Spine examination: The patient's cervical collar was removed. He has no tenderness to palpation of the cervical spine whatsoever.

The x-rays of the cervical spine, as well as the CT scan of the cervical spine, were reviewed. No fractures or subluxations are noted. CT scan of the head was reviewed, and it is negative for any intracranial pathology.

IMPRESSION/PLAN: In summary, we have a 17-year-old male involved in a motor vehicle accident. He has a mild concussive head injury, as evidenced by his amnesia, and I believe he did lose consciousness for a brief period; however, the exact amount of time for his loss of consciousness is unknown. There is no evidence of any cervical spine injury. The patient is neurologically normal. He does not need to wear a cervical collar. I explained to him and his mother, Gloria, that if the patient develops any weakness, numbness, or tingling in the arms or legs, trouble with his balance, sleepiness, vomiting, weakness of one side of the body, or any other symptoms, they should call their physician immediately.

I want to thank Dr. White for asking me to see this patient.

CPT Code(s): ____________________

ICD-10-CM Code(s): ____________________

ICD-9-CM Code(s): ____________________

Abstracting Questions

1. What items of Review of Systems (ROS) are documented? ____________________
2. Under what report heading(s) are the ROS found? ____________________
3. Was the patient the driver or passenger in the motor vehicle? ____________________

Case 1-11: Neurosurgery Consultation, Neck Pain

NEUROSURGERY CONSULTATION

Assign an E code to indicate how the injury occurred.

LOCATION: Inpatient, Hospital

PATIENT: MaryLou Robertson

ATTENDING PHYSICIAN: Rolando Ortez, MD

CONSULTANT: Timothy Pleasant, MD

REASON FOR REFERRAL: Neck pain.

HISTORY: This is a 12-year-old female who was doing a backward handstand and reportedly fell and injured her neck. She has had intermittent tingling in the left wrist and left ankle and once on the right wrist since this happened. Right now her tingling has resolved. She does not admit to having had any weakness or numbness at any point. She was admitted to the hospital last night when cervical spine x-rays showed a questionable subluxation at C2 and C3. The patient has had stable vital signs throughout. Her neurologic examination on admission was reportedly normal. Neurosurgery was asked to consult.

PAST MEDICAL HISTORY
1. She had chickenpox at age 4.
2. Immunizations are up to date.

MEDICATIONS: None.

SOCIAL HISTORY: She lives in Anytown with her mother and stepfather.

NEUROLOGIC EXAMINATION: The patient is awake, alert, and fully oriented. Cranial nerves are grossly intact. Motor examination is normal in the upper and lower extremities. Her sensory examination is intact to light touch in the upper and lower extremities. Her reflexes are normal and symmetric at the biceps, triceps, and brachioradialis. Her knee jerks and ankle jerks are normal and symmetric. Plantar responses are flexor. Her gait is normal. She can walk on her toes and heels. She can tandem walk.

RADIOLOGIC STUDIES: Her cervical spine x-ray shows probably physiologic subluxation of C2 on C3. Flexion and extension films were inadequate due to muscle spasm.

IMPRESSION/PLAN: In summary, we have a 12-year-old girl who was admitted with a questionable neck injury. I believe she has some musculoskeletal injury to the neck, but I believe her apparent subluxation of C2 on C3 is physiologic in nature. The patient should wear a cervical collar for a week, and the flexion and extension x-rays should be repeated until she can give adequate effort. The patient's pain is minimal at the present time, so there is no need for muscle relaxants or painkillers. I will see the patient as an outpatient in one week.

I want to thank Dr. Ortez for asking me to see this patient.

CPT Code(s): ______________________________

ICD-10-CM Code(s): ______________________________

ICD-9-CM Code(s): ______________________________

Abstracting Questions

1. Would the 1995 or 1997 Documentation Guidelines result in the highest level for this service?

   ____

Case 1-12: Neurosurgery Consultation, Leg Pain

NEUROSURGERY CONSULTATION

LOCATION: Inpatient, Hospital

PATIENT: Loren Schultz

ATTENDING PHYSICIAN: Frank Gaul, MD

CONSULTANT: Timothy Pleasant, MD

REASON FOR REFERRAL: Right leg pain.

HISTORY: This is a 50-year-old male who has had severe pain radiating down his right leg for one week. He tells me he was driving a lawnmower, cutting grass when he first experienced this pain. It has become worse over the last week, and he has noted a marked weakness in the right foot. The pain is in the right hip and radiates down the leg. The patient cannot say exactly where in the leg the pain radiates. He tells me it radiates throughout the whole right leg and right thigh. He also complains of numbness along the lateral aspect of the right calf and the back of the right thigh. Standing up is difficult. He describes the pain as an "electric shock." He went to the emergency room, and they gave him pain pills, but this did not help. He has tried physical therapy, but this has not helped either. He was unable to go to church last Sunday. He also admits to marked numbness in the right leg. He was admitted to the hospital three days ago. Walking is extremely difficult. Physical therapy has not helped. The painkillers have not helped. He tells me that when he walks, his foot goes sideways. He denies any bowel or bladder symptoms.

MEDICATIONS
1. Amaryl 4 mg q.d.
2. Aspirin.
3. Multivitamin.
4. Muscle relaxants and narcotics p.r.n. for this pain.

ALLERGIES: None known.

REVIEWS OF SYSTEMS AND PAST MEDICAL HISTORY: Significant for a nodule that was removed from his lung. He has a history of diabetes and is status post endarterectomy.

PAST SURGICAL HISTORY: He has had a right partial lung resection, gallbladder removal, and prostate surgery.

SOCIAL HISTORY: Noncontributory to the present problem.

FAMILY HISTORY: Noncontributory to the present problem.

EXAMINATION: Vital signs: He is afebrile. Blood pressure 135/80. Pulse 98. Respirations are unlabored. Neurologically, the patient's muscle strength in the lower extremities shows marked weakness of the anterior tibialis muscle and extensor hallucis longus muscle on the right side compatible with L5 nerve root weakness. His anterior tibialis and extensor hallucis longus would be graded 4/5. The strength in the left lower extremity is normal. Sensory examination shows decreased sensation to light touch over the right lateral calf and the right posterior thigh. Reflexes are hypoactive but symmetric at the knees and ankles. Straight leg raising test is positive on the right side at 30°C; this reproduces pain down the right leg. It is negative on the left side.

RADIOLOGIC STUDIES: An MRI of the lumbar spine shows L4-5 herniated disc with inferior migration with marked compression of the right L5 nerve root. There is also a bulge at the L5-S1 disc space on the right side, but I believe the disc fragment has broken off from the L4-5 space. The spinal alignment is normal and anatomical.

IMPRESSION/PLAN: In summary, we have a 50-year-old male with severe right leg pain. His neurologic examination shows motor and sensory changes compatible with a right L5 radiculopathy. His MRI scan shows a right L4-5 herniated disc with inferior migration with compression of the right L5 nerve root. I believe this patient has already sustained nerve damage, as is evidenced by the severe footdrop. I believe he is a candidate for surgery. It is unlikely this large disc fragment, which was broken off in the spinal canal, will resolve with medication or with time. The patient is reluctant to undergo surgery and wants to go to New Jersey and have a nerve specialist evaluate him. He tells me these nerve specialists are neither physicians nor chiropractors, but are able to manipulate his back in such a way to treat his problem. He is adamant about this. I explained to him that I am concerned about his nerve damage, but he wants to follow up with the nerve specialists in New Jersey. We will honor his wishes, and we will attempt to transfer his records there at his request.

I want to thank Dr. Gaul for asking me to see this patient, and I will continue to follow and monitor. Ultimately, he will need a physical therapy consult and an AFO orthosis for his footdrop. I am not optimistic at all that his symptoms will resolve short of surgical intervention. Again, I want to thank Dr. Gaul for the consult.

CPT Code(s): ____________________

ICD-10-CM Code(s): ____________________

ICD-9-CM Code(s): ____________________

Abstracting Questions

1. If the patient returns the following week to see Dr. Pleasant in his office to discuss/schedule a surgical procedure, would that visit be reportable? ____________________
2. With what code range would you report the return visit? ____________________

Case 1-13: Consultation, Intracerebral Hematoma

NEUROSURGERY CONSULTATION

LOCATION: Inpatient, Hospital

PATIENT: Mary Karr

ATTENDING PHYSICIAN: Ronald Green, MD

CONSULTANT: Timothy Pleasant, MD

The patient was seen in the emergency room. She was referred from Anytown. She has a large intracerebral hematoma, right temporal region. This could be a spontaneous bleed, it could be a traumatic bleed, or it could be an aneurysm. She is still moving all of her extremities. She is intubated and struggling. We will sedate her and have Dr. Dawson take over the medical management. We will go for an angiogram. If there is no aneurysm, go ahead and evacuate the clot.

CPT Code(s): ______________________________

ICD-10-CM Code(s): ______________________________

ICD-9-CM Code(s): ______________________________

Abstracting Questions

1. Location is listed as inpatient hospital, but the documentation indicates the patient was seen in the emergency department. What code range would be used to report this service? ______________________________
2. Are all three key components documented in this note? ______________________________

Case 1-14: Rehabilitation Consultation, Back Pain and SOB

REHABILITATION CONSULTATION

LOCATION: Inpatient, Hospital

PATIENT: Carlos Cano

ATTENDING PHYSICIAN: James Noonar, MD

CONSULTANT: Mary Barneswell, MD

The patient is a 59-year-old male who was admitted to the rehabilitation center 4 months ago with sudden onset of back pain and shortness of breath. He has a history of chronic obstructive pulmonary disease. Workup revealed congestive heart failure and atrial fibrillation. Back pain was believed to be secondary to cholesterol emboli. A CT scan of the lumbar spine showed degenerative changes only.

The patient's hospital course has been fairly stable otherwise. The back pain has improved. He has been participating in therapies, and rehabilitation medicine has been consulted to determine if he could benefit from comprehensive rehab program.

PAST MEDICAL/SURGICAL HISTORY: Please see previous notes.

SOCIAL HISTORY: The patient is married. He lives in Anytown in an apartment on the second floor. There is an elevator available, but the elevator is not too functional. Wife is in fair health and can assist him when he goes home. He does have a son, who lives in Denver, and a daughter, who lives in Orlando.

FUNCTIONAL HISTORY: Prior to admission he was able to ambulate by himself. He used no device. He does not drive; wife drives.

He is ambulating about 125 feet using a walker with assist. He transfers independently.

REVIEW OF SYSTEMS: He wears glasses. He denies the use of hearing aids or dentures. He denies any swallowing problems. He denies any chest pain, but does not deny shortness of breath. He is on about 3.5 liters of oxygen via the nasal cannula. He has a cough. He denies any nausea, emesis, or abdominal pain. He is voiding and moving bowels.

He denies any lower limb pain, weakness, or numbness. Back pain, he reports, generally worse with standing and walking. Overall, back pain has improved. Back pain is in the upper lumbar area/lower thoracic area. He has had no prior episodes of back pain that was as intense as it was when he came into the hospital.

PHYSICAL EXAMINATION: Pleasant 59-year-old white male, overweight, in no acute distress, and cooperative. Vital signs: Stable. He answers questions and follows commands appropriately. Skin: Warm and dry. HEENT: Head: Normocephalic. Eyes: Pupils equal and round. Visual acuity grossly normal. Ears: Hearing to spoken word is normal. Nose: Midline. Mouth and throat: Tongue is midline. Neck: Supple. No lymphadenopathy. Heart: Faint heart sounds auscultated. Lungs: Grossly clear bilaterally. Abdomen: Soft and nontender. Bowel sounds positive. Abdomen is slightly distended. Genitourinary: Not examined today. Extremities: Upper: Tone normal. Active range of motion at the shoulders is functional. Manual muscle testing reveals normal strength in the shoulders, triceps, biceps, and good grip. Lower: Passive range of motion at the knees is normal. Tone is normal. He can lift his limbs off the bed. Quads, hamstrings, ankle strength, and EHL normal. Neurologic: Cranial nerves II-XII grossly intact. Sensation intact to light touch, upper and lowers grossly. Reflexes in the lowers reveal patella 2/4, Achilles, not appreciated. Coordination of uppers reveal finger-to-finger movement; shows some moderate dysmetria bilaterally.

IMPRESSION
1. A 59-year-old male with general debility.
2. Improving thoracolumbar spine pain.
3. Coronary artery disease.
4. Chronic obstructive pulmonary disease.
5. History of chronic atrial fibrillation.
6. Hypertension.

PLAN: The patient may be a candidate for the comprehensive rehab program. Therapy evaluations are ongoing. Staff will follow and make further recommendations as needed.

CPT Code(s): ______________________________

ICD-10-CM Code(s): ______________________________

ICD-9-CM Code(s): ______________________________

Abstracting Questions

1. What chronic condition(s) is/are in the patient's past medical history? ______________________________
2. Do these chronic conditions have a bearing on the current treatment plan? ______________________________

Case 1-15: Urology Consultation, Oliguria

UROLOGY CONSULTATION

LOCATION: Inpatient, Hospital

PATIENT: Sally Scheel

ATTENDING PHYSICIAN: Frank Gaul, MD

CONSULTANT: Ira Avila, MD

REASON FOR CONSULTATION: Request of Dr. Gaul regarding oliguria, increasing BUN and creatinine.

HISTORY: This is an 82-year-old woman who I previously have known because of her husband who had prostate CA. She has been hospitalized here with a picture of increasing peripheral edema, decreasing urinary output, and increasing BUN and creatinine. She has gotten to the point of this scenario that there is a real question of doing dialysis. Her most recent creatinine is 5.4. She has an interesting history at this point.

Basically, this lady has, over the course of the past months, been noted to have an increasing level of creatinine. Her family doctor has been watching that with her. She has had increasing edema as well. Along the way she has had an ultrasound that shows a very thin-walled, probably nonfunctioning right kidney. A very mild amount of hydronephrosis was noted on the left side. No renogram has been performed. No CT scan has been performed in order to evaluate possible reasons for obstruction. The patient underwent bilateral renal stent placement through the ureters in retrograde fashion. These were initially placed in October, and with increasing peripheral edema, her stents were re-replaced again just recently at the beginning of this month. Despite this, the patient has continued to have an elevating creatinine situation, and she has been on a load of medications, which have also been somewhat renally toxic and which have been discontinued. These include Demadex and triamterene.

Currently, I have been asked by Dr. Gaul to see the patient to evaluate whether there is anything that I can do to help her with outlet obstruction phenomenon.

PAST MEDICAL HISTORY
1. History of hypertension.
2. She is status post breast removal for breast carcinoma.
3. She has a history of asthma.
4. She has had a prior cholecystectomy.
5. Bilateral mastectomies.
6. Appendectomy.
7. Varicose vein stripping.
8. She has a known history of gastroesophageal reflux problems.

MEDICATIONS
1. Maxair.
2. Vasotec.
3. Protonix.
4. Theophylline.
5. Demadex.
6. Triamterene.
7. Slo-Bid.

ALLERGIES: No known medication allergies.

HABITS: She has never used tobacco. Alcohol intake has been very minimal.

SOCIAL HISTORY: She is widowed. She has been a homemaker. Her husband had prostate cancer, and I took care of him through that issue.

FAMILY HISTORY: Not noted exclusively. Apparently she is the last in her line. Her mom and dad died in their 50s of unknown illness. There has been no known real cancer/cardiovascular disease in her family.

REVIEW OF SYSTEMS: Noted and consistent with weight gain under constitutional change. Respiratory: She has had shortness of breath secondary to ongoing asthma. Cardiovascular: She has had some palpitations. Rapid heartbeat. This has been checked by cardiology. Cutaneous status is negative. Breasts negative because of prior mastectomies. She denies any hematologic, lymphatic, or neurologic problems. Endocrine: Thirsty. Musculoskeletal: Diffuse arthritis. Gastrointestinal: Constipation. Reflux disease. Genitourinary: Voiding normally but in smaller than normal amounts.

PHYSICAL EXAMINATION: Healthy-looking 82-year-old lady who is lying in bed; she is very edematous looking. She is alert and oriented times three. Friendly and talkative. Vital signs: Blood pressure 140/61. Pulse 90. Respiratory rate 20. Abdomen: Upper abdominal examination is slightly obese. Evidence of surgical incisions that are well healed. No specific masses. She is a little bit tympanitic, but there is no evidence of any major rebound tenderness or changes to the abdominal wall or cavity. Lower abdominal wall is also normal. No flank pain or discomfort. Suprapubic: A soft Foley catheter exiting the urethra appears normal in size, unremarkable. Small amount of amber urine present. Legs and buttocks: Massively swollen, 2–3+ pitting edema along the presacral areas posteriorly. Labial pitting edema is noted. Vaginal vault is stenotic. Hypoestrogenic-type changes. Foley catheter exiting with a normal meatus. No palpable masses along the urethra, etc. She has not had a prior hysterectomy. We are unable to visualize the cervix or do an adequate bimanual examination because of discomfort, stenosis, and swelling. No obvious cystocele or rectocele present.

IMPRESSION: Marked hydronephrosis of the right kidney. This is probably a congenital process, with known history of small dense kidney on the left side with probable prerenal disease. No further hydronephrosis is noted on the review of the most recent ultrasound.

PLAN: The patient is going to go on to get a catheter for dialysis. It might be wise at this point to do a CT scan on her at some point in the next few days just to look for any retroperitoneal disease or other causes for potential bilateral ureteral obstruction.

CPT Code(s): ______________________________

ICD-10-CM Code(s): ______________________________

ICD-9-CM Code(s): ______________________________

Abstracting Questions

1. What part of the documentation indicates oliguria? ______________________________

Case 1-16: Thoracic Medicine/Critical Care Progress Note, Lung Cancer

THORACIC MEDICINE/CRITICAL CARE PROGRESS NOTE

LOCATION: Inpatient, Hospital

PATIENT: Ellen Zutz

ATTENDING PHYSICIAN: Gregory Dawson, MD

This patient has been hospitalized for the past week with primary tumor of the middle lobe of the right lung. She also has COPD asthma. The patient requires 4 liter/min while walking, as shown by a walking O_2 desaturation study. Po_2 today on room air was 58. For somebody with heart disease and prone to congestive heart failure, we will leave her on 1 liter/min when she is awake and asleep, and 4 liter/min when she is walking. We will check in about 2 weeks to see if she has lost the need for this.

CPT Code(s): ____________________

ICD-10-CM Code(s): ____________________

ICD-9-CM Code(s): ____________________

Abstracting Questions

1. Does the documentation meet the criteria to be reported as critical care? ____________________

Case 1-17: Clinic Visit, Diarrhea

CLINIC NOTE

FOLLOW-UP CLINIC VISIT

SUBJECTIVE: This is a 3½-year-old girl who presents today. Mother states that patient has had diarrhea over the past 3-4 days. Yesterday she had about 4–5 stools. They have been mustard colored, real runny, sometimes in little slivers. No blood has been present. She threw up 3-4 days ago, but this has since ended. Her eating is down, although she is drinking a lot. She will complain of her stomach hurting. Her temperature was as high as 103°F, and that was about 3 days ago. She is taking Motrin.

OBJECTIVE: On general appearance: She is alert and does not appear to be in any acute distress. Temperature is 97.2°F. Weight is 42 pounds. HEENT: Eyes are clear. The right TM has some increased erythema present. Landmarks are still seen. The left TM is nice and clear with good landmarks. Oropharynx is unremarkable. Neck is supple. Heart reveals a regular rate and rhythm without murmur. GU: Normal female genitalia.

ASSESSMENT
1. Viral gastroenteritis.
2. Possibly early right otitis media.

PLAN: I did discuss with mother that we could put her daughter on an antibiotic now, but we also could wait to see if she starts complaining of right ear pain or if her fever comes back. If that is the case, I did give mother a prescription for Amoxicillin to have her daughter take 375 mg p.o. t.i.d. × 10 days, and I would want to recheck her ear in 3 weeks. If she does not have any complaints or fever, mother will hold off just so Amoxicillin does not worsen her diarrhea. Mother was in agreement with this plan.

CPT Code(s): ______________________________

ICD-10-CM Code(s): ______________________________

ICD-9-CM Code(s): ______________________________

Abstracting Questions

1. What category of E/M codes is used to report this service? ______________________________
2. What body system is reviewed in the statement “right TM”? ______________________________

Case 1-18: Cardiology Consultation, Chest Pain and SOB

CARDIOLOGY CONSULTATION

LOCATION: Outpatient, Clinic

PATIENT: Mary Blane

PRIMARY CARE PHYSICIAN: Ronald Green, MD

CARDIOLOGY CONSULTANT: James Elhart, MD

CHIEF COMPLAINT: Chest pain and shortness of breath.

HISTORY OF PRESENT ILLNESS: This is a 46-year-old female who says that for the past couple of months she has had progressive shortness of breath. She is short of breath when she walks between one and two blocks. She also has experienced exertional chest tightness and is diaphoretic. Rest relieves the discomfort for about 10 to 15 minutes.

CARDIAC RISK FACTORS: Only cigarette smoking and dyslipidemia.

PAST MEDICAL HISTORY: She is married. She used to smoke a pack of cigarettes a day for 10 years. Currently, she smokes 7 to 10 cigarettes a week. She has been a smoker for 23 years. The patient does not drink alcohol.

FAMILY HISTORY: Father had myocardial infarction in his 40s and died from myocardial infarction in his 80s.

CURRENT MEDICATIONS: Aleve.

ALLERGIES: None.

PHYSICAL EXAMINATION: Very pleasant female who appears to be in no acute distress. Blood pressure is 112/70. Pulse is 80. Neck is supple without JVD or bruit. Lungs are clear to auscultation and percussion. Heart: Regular S1 and S2; no S3 or S4. Abdomen is soft and nontender. Bowel sounds are well heard. Patient is alert and oriented.

Electrocardiogram is within normal limits.

ASSESSMENT
1. Chest pain; etiology is not clear.
2. Shortness of breath.
3. History of dyslipidemia.

RECOMMENDATION
1. Echocardiogram.
2. Persantine Cardiolite stress test.
3. Further management will be determined by the results of these investigations. Meanwhile, the patient will rest, take daily aspirin, and was given a prescription for sublingual nitroglycerin.

CPT Code(s): ______________________________

ICD-10-CM Code(s): ______________________________

ICD-9-CM Code(s): ______________________________

Abstracting Questions

1. Has the consultant completed his evaluation of this patient? ____________________

2. If the patient returns to see Dr. Elhart, what category of codes would report the visit? ____________________

Case 1-19: Clinic Visit, Abdominal Pain

CLINIC NOTE

FOLLOW-UP CLINIC VISIT

SUBJECTIVE: This is a 26-year-old white female, gravida 4, para 2, in today with complaints of right lower quadrant pain since early this morning. She states that when she first woke up, she had noticed that her abdomen was quite tender. The pain then centered in the right lower quadrant. She has complained of chills all day and has been wearing an extra sweater. She did have an adequate bowel movement this morning without pain on bowel movement. She has a history of a hysterectomy, but she did not have an oophorectomy. She has requested to be evaluated for right lower quadrant pain.

ALLERGIES: None.

OBJECTIVE: Stat CBC was done, which did not show any increased lymphocytes or differential shift. Hemoglobin was low at 11.3. Pelvic ultrasound did not show any abnormalities in the appendix area. Bladder was not filled, so no evaluation of ovaries was done. Pelvic exam showed cervical stub is in place in the vagina. No adnexal masses were noted. Cervix was freely mobile. Abdomen was quite firm to palpation and percussion.

ASSESSMENT: Right lower quadrant pain.

PLAN: Reassured. Reviewed the differential diagnosis symptoms between appendicitis, ovarian cyst formation, and gastroenteritis. Advised that she continue with high-fiber foods and increase fluids to decrease symptoms.

CPT Code(s): ______________________________

ICD-10-CM Code(s): ______________________________

ICD-9-CM Code(s): ______________________________

Abstracting Questions

1. The visit is listed as a "follow-up" clinic visit. The patient presents with a new problem. What category of codes is appropriate? ______________________________
2. Was there a definitive diagnosis? ______________________________

Chapter 2
Anesthesiology

Make sure to check evolve for the latest content updates

Case 2-1: Perforated Appendicitis

Assign anesthesia code(s) and any necessary modifiers. Do not assign surgery codes. Do not assign diagnosis codes. During this procedure the anesthesiologist was medically directing two CRNAs providing anesthesia for concurrent procedures. The patient's physical status is P2.

OPERATIVE REPORT

LOCATION: Inpatient, Hospital

PATIENT: Laurence Hooper

ATTENDING PHYSICIAN: Gary Sanchez, MD

SURGEON: Gary Sanchez, MD

PREOPERATIVE DIAGNOSIS: Perforated appendicitis.

POSTOPERATIVE DIAGNOSIS: Same.

ANESTHESIA: General.

ANESTHESIOLOGIST: Janice E. Larson, MD

PROCEDURE: The patient was brought to the operating room, placed under general anesthesia, and prepped and draped sterilely. The patient's advanced age is a concern, since he is 92. A right lower quadrant skin incision was made with a #10 blade, and dissection was carried down through the subcutaneous tissue using electrocautery. The anterior sheath of the rectus fascia was opened. The rectus was retracted medially. The posterior sheath and peritoneum were grasped with curved clamps and sharply incised, allowing entry into the peritoneal cavity. There were a few adhesions, which we took down sharply. We then delivered the appendix up and into the wound. We took down the mesoappendix between Kelly clamps and tied the vascular pedicles with 2–0 silk free ties. The base of the appendix was then crushed. It was tied with 0 Vicryl. It was inverted into the base of the cecum with a 3–0 silk pursestring suture. The abdomen was then irrigated with saline until returns were clear. We closed the posterior sheath and peritoneum with running 0 Vicryl, closed the anterior sheath with interrupted 0 Vicryl, and closed the skin with subcuticular 4–0 undyed Vicryl. Steri-Strips and sterile Band-Aids were applied. All sponge and needle counts were correct. Before the patient left the operating room, the wound was anesthetized with a total of 30 cc of 0.50% Sensorcaine with epinephrine solution.

CPT Code(s): ______________________________

Abstracting Questions

1. What is the main term referenced in the index of the CPT to locate the code?
   ____
2. What was the subterm used in the CPT index to locate the anesthesia code? ______________
3. Does the quadrant entered to perform the surgical procedure affect CPT anesthesia code assignment? ________
4. Was the procedure at the abdominal wall or intraperitoneal? ______________
5. Were there any Qualifying Circumstances to report? ______________
6. Who decides what Physical Status Modifier should be reported? ______________
7. Was the anesthesiologist providing service or medically directing cases? ______________

Case 2-2: Right Inguinal Herniorrhaphy

Assign anesthesia code(s) only. Do not assign surgery codes. Do not assign diagnosis codes. The anesthesiologist was medically directing three CRNAs concurrently. The patient's physical status is P2.

OPERATIVE REPORT

LOCATION: Outpatient, Hospital

PATIENT: Gary Holter

ATTENDING PHYSICIAN: Gary Sanchez, MD

SURGEON: Gary Sanchez, MD

PREOPERATIVE DIAGNOSIS: Right inguinal hernia.

POSTOPERATIVE DIAGNOSIS: Same.

PROCEDURE PERFORMED: Right inguinal herniorrhaphy.

ANESTHESIA: General.

ANESTHESIOLOGIST: Janice E. Larson, MD

PROCEDURE: This 45-year-old patient was brought to the operating room, placed under general anesthesia, and prepped and draped sterilely. A right groin skin incision was made with a #10 blade. Dissection was carried down through the subcutaneous tissues using electrocautery. The external oblique was identified and opened along the length of its fibers along the external ring. Spermatic cord was identified and looped with a Penrose drain. Hernia sac was dissected free. High ligation was then performed with a 3–0 Vicryl suture ligature and a 2–0 silk free tie. The patulous internal ring was then closed with a simple interrupted 3–0 Vicryl suture. The floor of the canal looked quite good. We then closed the external oblique with a running 3–0 Vicryl, and Scarpa's with interrupted 3–0 Vicryl, and closed the skin with subcuticular 4–0 undyed Vicryl. Steri-Strips and sterile Band-Aids were applied. All sponge and needle counts were correct. Patient tolerated the procedure well and was taken to the recovery room in stable condition.

CPT Code(s): ______________________________

Abstracting Questions

1. What area of the body was repaired? ______________________________
2. Does the type (inguinal) affect the CPT anesthesia code assignment? ______________________________
3. Does the age of the patient affect the CPT anesthesia code? ______________________________
4. What, if any, qualifying circumstance was reported? ______________________________

Case 2-3: Laparoscopic Cholecystectomy

Assign anesthesia code(s) only. Do not assign surgery codes. Do not assign diagnosis codes. The anesthesiologist personally performed this service. The patient's physical status is P3 as he has uncontrolled hypertension.

OPERATIVE REPORT

LOCATION: Outpatient, Hospital

PATIENT: Mable Moore

ATTENDING PHYSICIAN: Gary Sanchez, MD

SURGEON: Gary Sanchez, MD

PREOPERATIVE DIAGNOSIS: Symptomatic cholelithiasis.

POSTOPERATIVE DIAGNOSIS: Same.

PROCEDURE PERFORMED: Laparoscopic cholecystectomy.

ANESTHESIA: General.

ANESTHESIOLOGIST: Janice E. Larson, MD

PROCEDURE: The patient was brought to the operating room, placed under general anesthesia, and prepped and draped sterilely after a Foley catheter and oral gastric tubes were inserted. The patient has severe hypertension, which is a concern. Supraumbilical skin incision was made with a #11 blade, and dissection was carried down through subcutaneous tissues bluntly. Midline fascia was grasped with Kocher clamp. A 0 Vicryl suture was then placed on either side of the midline fascia. A Veress needle was inserted into the abdominal cavity. A drop test confirmed placement within the peritoneal space. The abdomen was then insufflated with carbon dioxide. A 10-mm trocar port and laparoscope were introduced, showing no damage to the overlying viscera. Under direct vision, three additional trocar ports were placed: one upper midline 10 mm and two right upper quadrant 5 mm. The gallbladder was grasped and elevated from its fossa. The cystic duct and artery were dissected free, doubly clipped proximally and distally before dividing them with the hook scissors. The gallbladder was then shelled from its fossa using electrocautery and brought up and out of the upper midline incision. The abdomen was irrigated with saline until returns were clear. Trocar ports were then removed under direct vision with no evidence of bleeding. Supraumbilical port site fascial defect was closed with a single interrupted 0 Vicryl suture. The skin at all port sites was closed with subcuticular 4–0 undyed Vicryl. Steri-Strips and sterile Band-Aids were applied. All sponge and needle counts were correct. The patient tolerated the procedure well and was taken to the recovery in stable condition.

CPT Code(s): ______________________________

Abstracting Questions

1. Does the laparoscopic approach affect code selection? ______________________
2. Was a physical status modifier required? ______________________
3. Was the anesthesiologist providing service or medically directing cases? ______________________

Case 2-4: Left Breast Biopsy

Assign anesthesia code(s) only. Do not assign surgery codes. Do not assign diagnosis codes. The patient's physical status is P1.

OPERATIVE REPORT

LOCATION: Outpatient, Hospital

PATIENT: Adrienne Gardener

ATTENDING PHYSICIAN: Gary Sanchez, MD

SURGEON: Gary Sanchez, MD

PREOPERATIVE DIAGNOSIS: Left breast mass.

POSTOPERATIVE DIAGNOSIS: Same.

PROCEDURE PERFORMED: Left breast biopsy.

ANESTHESIA: Local with IV sedation and monitored anesthesia care.

ANESTHESIOLOGIST: Janice E. Larson, MD

PROCEDURE: The patient was brought to the operating room, given IV sedation, and then anesthetized with a total of 30 cc of 1% Sensorcaine with epinephrine solution. Incision was made over the top of the mass with a #15 blade, and dissection was carried down through subcutaneous tissues sharply. We encountered the mass, which appeared to be a fibroadenoma. We excised this sharply. We got the entire lesion. We controlled bleeding with electrocautery. We then closed the skin with subcuticular 4–0 undyed Vicryl. Steri-Strips and sterile Band-Aids were applied. She tolerated this well and was taken to recovery room in stable condition.

Pathology Report Later Indicated: Fibroadenoma.

CPT Code(s): ____________________

Abstracting Questions

1. Do you report the sedation with CPT anesthesia codes or medicine codes? ____________________
2. Was the procedure superficial (subcutaneous) or deep (internal structures)? ____________________

Case 2-5: Amputation

Assign anesthesia code(s) only. Do not assign surgery codes. Do not assign diagnosis codes. The patient's physical status is P3.

OPERATIVE REPORT

LOCATION: Inpatient, Hospital

PATIENT: Lee Laetrile

ATTENDING PHYSICIAN: Gary Sanchez, MD

SURGEON: Gary Sanchez, MD

ANESTHESIA: General.

ANESTHESIOLOGIST: Janice E. Larson, MD

PREOPERATIVE DIAGNOSIS: Necrotic left foot, gangrenous.

POSTOPERATIVE DIAGNOSIS: Same.

PROCEDURE PERFORMED: Left above-knee amputation.

PROCEDURE: The patient was brought to the operating theater and placed in the supine position on the operating room table. After receiving a general anesthetic, he was prepped and draped in a sterile fashion. A fish-mouth incision was marked out on the left leg above the knee. Incisions were made. He has a fair amount of varicosities. These were rather ropey, large varicosities on his thigh. Most of these were on the medial aspect. After being transected, the varicosities were ligated by clamps and then 3–0 Vicryl ties or 3–0 Vicryl stick ties. There was some blood loss with this. He had a very edematous leg. There was also a lot of edema in the leg, which, of course, came out of the tissues. Sharp dissection was carried down through the subcutaneous tissues all the way through the fascia and through the muscles. It came down onto the femur. This was cleared off. We used a right-angle clamp to get around the superficial femoral artery and vein. These were clamped with Lahey right angles, transected, then ligated with 2–0 Vicryl. Proximally it was double ligated with a 2–0 Vicryl free tie and then a 2–0 silk stick tie. A periosteal elevator was used on the femur. This was taken back to about 10 cm from the proximal condyles. I wanted to be sure that we had made our incision such that we would be slightly more proximal than typical. Patient has had a minor problem with healing of his right leg, but this has basically held up. The left leg also is a concern for being able to heal, and so I wanted to be sure we were proximal enough so we could promote healing. The femur was transected with a Gigli saw. I then used a guillotine knife to transect the posterior muscle group. Clamps were applied to the bleeding vessels. This included the popliteal artery, which had already been transected and ligated. The sciatic nerve was infiltrated with 0.5% Marcaine with epinephrine. I then retracted and clamped it proximally, then transected and ligated with a 2–0 Vicryl. Bleeding points in the muscles were oversewn with 3–0 Vicryl stick ties. The end of the bone was smoothed with a bone rasp. The wound was then irrigated with 3 liters of kanamycin/Bacitracin in LF. The Ortholav was used for this. Surgicel was then applied into the open end of the femur in the bone marrow cavity. A 10-mm flat Jackson-Pratt drain was also placed and brought out through a separate stab wound laterally. We then closed the fascia and the muscles together using interrupted sutures of 2–0 Vicryl. The skin was then brought together with staples. Xeroform, fluffs, Kerlix, and an Ace wrap were then applied. The patient tolerated the procedure well and went to the recovery room in stable condition. I met with the patient's family postoperatively to discuss the operative findings.

CPT Code(s): ____________________

Abstracting Questions

1. What was the level of amputation? ____________________

Case 2-6: Umbilical Herniorrhaphy

Assign anesthesia code(s) only. Do not assign surgery codes. Do not assign diagnosis codes. The patient's physical status is P1.

OPERATIVE REPORT

LOCATION: Outpatient, Hospital

PATIENT: Ben Bolten

ATTENDING PHYSICIAN: Gary Sanchez, MD

SURGEON: Gary Sanchez, MD

PREOPERATIVE DIAGNOSIS: Umbilical hernia.

POSTOPERATIVE DIAGNOSIS: Same.

PROCEDURE PERFORMED: Umbilical herniorrhaphy.

ANESTHESIA: General.

ANESTHESIOLOGIST: Janice E. Larson, MD

PROCEDURE: This 53-year-old patient was brought to the operating room and placed under general anesthesia, then prepped and draped sterilely. An infraumbilical skin incision was made with a #15 blade. Dissection was carried down through subcutaneous tissues using electrocautery. The hernia sac was dissected free from the umbilicus and reduced. The fascial defect was then closed with interrupted 0 Vicryl sutures. The umbilicus was tacked back down to the fascia with a 3–0 undyed Vicryl, and skin was closed with subcuticular 4–0 undyed Vicryl. Steri-Strips and sterile bandage were applied. All sponge and needle counts were correct. Before patient left the operating room, the wound was anesthetized with a total of 30 cc of 0.5% Sensorcaine with epinephrine solution.

CPT Code(s): ______________________________

Abstracting Questions

1. What area of the body was repaired? ______________________________

Case 2-7: Takedown Colostomy and Cholecystectomy

Assign anesthesia code(s) only. Do not assign surgery codes. Do not assign diagnosis codes. The anesthesiologist was supervising two concurrent procedures. The patient's physical status is P2.

OPERATIVE REPORT

LOCATION: Inpatient, Hospital

PATIENT: Simon Sulten

ATTENDING PHYSICIAN: Gary Sanchez, MD

SURGEON: Gary Sanchez, MD

PREOPERATIVE DIAGNOSES
1. Colostomy for obstructing colon cancer.
2. Symptomatic cholelithiasis.

POSTOPERATIVE DIAGNOSES: Same.

PROCEDURE PERFORMED
1. Takedown colostomy with end-to-end colorectostomy.
2. Open cholecystectomy.

ANESTHESIA: General.

ANESTHESIOLOGIST: Janice E. Larson, MD

PROCEDURE: The patient was brought to the operating room, placed under general anesthesia, and prepped and draped sterilely. The previous midline was reopened with the #10 blade, and we excised the old scar. We carried out dissection through subcutaneous tissues using electrocautery. Midline fascia was divided sharply. We entered the peritoneal cavity and entered the midline fascia along the length of the incision. We took down numerous filmy adhesions and ran the small bowel from the terminal ileum to the ligament of Treitz, which appeared normal. First, we placed an Omni retractor and exposed the right upper quadrant. We identified the cystic duct and cystic artery and tied them off with 0 silk ties proximally and distally before transecting them. We then shelled the gallbladder from its fossa using electrocautery. We placed a pack up by the liver bed. We then identified the rectal stump and dissected this free. We then made an elliptical incision around the colostomy opening and carried our dissection down to fascia, freed up the stoma, and fired our TLC 75 stapler across the descending colon. We sent the specimen to pathology for permanent. We mobilized the left colon along the avascular line of Toldt up and around the splenic flexure. Once we had adequate length, we placed a Glassman clamp proximally on the rectum and distally on the descending colon. We then performed a two-layer, hand-sewn, end-to-end anastomosis with an outer layer of 3–0 silk Lembert and inner layer of running 3–0 Vicryl. There was a patent anastomosis, and we could easily milk contents through with no evidence of spilling. We then closed the fascia from the colostomy site with interrupted 0 Vicryl and running 0 PDS. We closed the skin with skin clips. All sponge and needle counts were correct. Patient tolerated this well and was taken to recovery in stable condition.

CPT Code(s): ______________________________

Abstracting Questions

1. Was a supervision modifier required? ______________________________

Case 2-8: Modified Radical Mastectomy

Assign anesthesia code(s) only. Do not assign surgery codes. Do not assign diagnosis codes. The patient's physical status is P1.

OPERATIVE REPORT

LOCATION: Inpatient, Hospital

PATIENT: Lucy Bates

ATTENDING PHYSICIAN: Gary Sanchez, MD

SURGEON: Gary Sanchez, MD

PREOPERATIVE DIAGNOSIS: Right breast cancer.

POSTOPERATIVE DIAGNOSIS: Same.

OPERATIVE PROCEDURE: Right modified radical mastectomy.

ANESTHESIA: General.

ANESTHESIOLOGIST: Janice E. Larson, MD

PROCEDURE: The patient was brought to the operating room, placed under general anesthesia, and prepped and draped sterilely. An elliptical incision was made around the right nipple to include the biopsy site, and flaps were created superiorly, inferiorly, medially, and laterally down to the pectoralis superiorly to the rectus fascia inferiorly, sternum medially, and latissimus laterally. We then took the breast off the pectoralis fascia and entered the axillary space. Perforating vessels were either cauterized or ligated with 3–0 Vicryl suture ligatures. We entered the axillary space. We could feel several lymph nodes. We excised the lymph nodes. We could see the thoracodorsal nerve easily and kept this free from our dissection. We were unable to identify the long thoracic nerve. Once we had stripped the lymph nodes free, we irrigated with saline. We could easily see the axillary vein superiorly, the latissimus dorsi laterally, and the pectoralis medially, and had cleaned all the lymph nodes out of this space. We then irrigated with sterile water and placed two Jackson-Pratt drains: a lateral drain going into the axilla, and a medial drain going underneath the skin flaps. We then closed in two layers with a deep layer of 3–0 Vicryl. Steri-Strips and sterile Band-Aids were applied. All sponge and needle counts were correct. Patient tolerated the procedure well and was taken to recovery in stable condition.

CPT Code(s): ______________________________

Abstracting Questions

1. Was a supervision modifier required? ______________________________

Case 2-9: Incision and Drainage of Perirectal Abscess

Assign anesthesia code(s) only. Do not assign surgery codes. Do not assign diagnosis codes. The patient's physical status is P3.

OPERATIVE REPORT

LOCATION: Outpatient, Hospital

PATIENT: Suzy Tarsinski

ATTENDING PHYSICIAN: Gary Sanchez, MD

SURGEON: Gary Sanchez, MD

PREOPERATIVE DIAGNOSIS: Perirectal abscess.

POSTOPERATIVE DIAGNOSIS: Same.

PROCEDURE PERFORMED: Incision and drainage of perirectal abscess.

ANESTHESIA: Spinal.

ANESTHESIOLOGIST: Janice E. Larson, MD

PROCEDURE: The patient was brought back to the operating room, and after a spinal anesthetic had been given, the area of the rectum was cleaned and draped in the usual fashion after the patient had been placed in a jackknife position. An incision was made over the top of this abscess with a #10-blade scalpel. We entered the abscessed cavity, which returned large amounts of purulent material. We broke up the loculations, debrided the necrotic tissue with a #10 blade, and irrigated with a liter of saline. We then were able to pack the cavity with sewed Kerlix. The patient tolerated the procedure well, and all sponges and needles were accounted for at the end of the procedure. Soon she could be transferred to the Post Anesthesia Care Unit in stable condition.

CPT Code(s): ____

Abstracting Questions

1. For the purpose of locating an anesthesia code in the CPT manual, what was the location of the I&D?

____

Case 2-10: Division and Insetting of Flap

Assign anesthesia code(s) only. Do not assign surgery codes. Do not assign diagnosis codes. Physical status is P2 for well-controlled diabetes.

OPERATIVE REPORT

LOCATION: Outpatient, Hospital

PATIENT: Leslie May

ATTENDING PHYSICIAN: Gary Sanchez, MD

SURGEON: Gary Sanchez, MD

PREOPERATIVE DIAGNOSIS: Status post thenar flap, right middle fingertip.

POSTOPERATIVE DIAGNOSIS: Status post thenar flap, right middle fingertip.

PROCEDURE PERFORMED: Division and insetting of thenar flap, right middle finger and palm.

ANESTHESIA: General.

PROCEDURE: The patient was brought to the operating room, and general anesthesia was induced. The right upper extremity was removed from the bandages. We prepped it with Betadine and draped it in sterile fashion. We then exsanguinated the limb, and a tourniquet was inflated to 250 mm Hg for 30 minutes. We then divided the flap. Attention was first directed to the thenar eminence. There was no sign of infection. The sutures were removed, and we lightly debrided some of the scarring. We then inset the flap and sutured this with interrupted 5–0 nylon suture. We then inspected the fingertip. All sutures were removed. The flap was viable. There was no sign of infection at the flap proximally. We inset the flap proximally and set this in with interrupted 5–0 nylon suture. The nail plate had elevated off the nailbed, and we therefore cleansed dried blood from underneath the nailbed. There was no sign of infection. We irrigated this with sterile saline. We then applied Xeroform over all wounds, and we placed a compression bandage across the palm and also TubeGauz bandage on the finger. Tourniquet was released, and good circulation returned to the hand.

The patient will be dismissed as an outpatient today with plans for follow-up back in the office in 7-10 days.

DISCHARGE MEDICATIONS: Darvocet-N 100, 30 tablets.

CPT Code(s): ______________________________

Abstracting Questions

1. The service provided was to what body system? ______________________________

Case 2-11: Intracerebral Hematoma

Assign anesthesia code(s) only. Do not assign surgery codes. Do not assign diagnosis codes. The patient is not expected to survive without this procedure.

OPERATIVE PROCEDURE

LOCATION: Inpatient, Hospital

PATIENT: Suzy Kunklemann

ATTENDING PHYSICIAN: Gary Sanchez, MD

SURGEON: Gary Sanchez, MD

PREOPERATIVE DIAGNOSIS: Intracerebral hematoma, right temporal lobe.

POSTOPERATIVE DIAGNOSIS: Intracerebral hematoma, right temporal lobe.

PROCEDURE PERFORMED: Osteoplastic craniotomy, right temporal area; evacuation of intracerebral hematoma.

ANESTHESIA: General.

PROCEDURE: This patient is not expected to survive without this procedure, and at this point we have no other choice but to proceed. Under general anesthesia, the patient's head was placed in the Mayfield pins. The right frontal temporoparietal area was prepped and draped in the usual manner. A linear incision was made extending from the midline of the temporal fossa up to the midportion of the scalp. The skin was incised. The temporalis muscle was separated and divided off the bone. I did a craniotomy here the size of a half dollar coin and made a burr hole. I utilized the craniotome to elevate the bone flap, which was a free bone flap. This was then removed. We placed the Weitlaners into the wound and then incised the dura in a cruciate fashion over the temporal lobe. I then entered the middle temple gyrus, irrigated much of the clot from the temporal and posterior parietal areas, and evacuated the clot from the area. This took copious irrigation. We used cotton balls for hemostasis. I did this numerous times until all the bleeders were coagulated. I then lined the cystic cavity with Gelfoam and coagulated the edges of the raw brain. I closed the dura with 4–0 Vicryl. This was closed in a watertight fashion. I used 2–0 Vicryl to elevate the dura to the bone flap with Wurzburg plates, two of them, using plates and screws. I then closed the scalp in one layer using 0 Vicryl on the temporalis muscle and fascia, and the skin was approximated with 2–0 nylon interrupted mattress sutures. Dressing was applied, and the patient was on the ventilator and discharged to the surgical intensive care unit.

CPT Code(s): ____________________

Abstracting Questions

1. Would a physical status modifier be required? ____________________

Chapter 3
Cardiology

Make sure to check evolve learning system for the latest content updates

Case 3-1: Catheter Placement

OPERATIVE REPORT

LOCATION: Inpatient, Hospital

PATIENT: Tim Luther

ATTENDING/ADMIT PHYSICIAN: Frank Gaul, MD

SURGEON: David Barton, MD

PREOPERATIVE DIAGNOSIS: Fluid overload state, no urine output, acute renal failure.

POSTOPERATIVE DIAGNOSIS: Fluid overload state, no urine output, acute renal failure.

PROCEDURE PERFORMED: Temporary dialysis catheter placement.

PROCEDURE: This 77-year-old patient was brought to the emergency room. The right femoral vein was selected. This was tried with the left IJ vein earlier without success. I reserved the right IJ for a central line that will be placed by interventional radiology in the morning. The right femoral vein was localized using ultrasound. *(The ultrasound is not a reportable service.)* The area was prepped in the usual fashion. One-percent lidocaine was used for local anesthesia. The right femoral vein was accessed under real-time ultrasound guidance without difficulty. The guidewire was advanced smoothly. The hook needle was taken out. The right femoral vein was dilated. An 11.5 French 16-cm temporary dialysis catheter with a straight extension was advanced through the right femoral vein over the guidewire using the Seldinger technique without difficulty. Both ports had good venous blood return. Both ports were flushed with saline and heparin. The catheter was secured to the skin. The patient tolerated the procedure very well without immediate complication. Dialysis will be done semi-urgently.

CPT Code(s): ______________________________

ICD-10-CM Code(s): ______________________________

ICD-9-CM Code(s): ______________________________

Abstracting Questions

1. What is another name for a catheter or central line? ______
2. What vessel was used for the access point for the catheter? ______
3. Was the insertion central or peripheral? ______
4. Was the catheter tunneled or non-tunneled? ______
5. Does the age of the patient affect code selection? ______
6. Was there a port and/or pump inserted? ______
7. Does the type of radiologic guidance affect the radiology code selection? ______

Case 3-2: Chart Note, Therapeutic Apheresis

LOCATION: Inpatient, Hospital

PATIENT: George Lightfoot

ATTENDING PHYSICIAN: George Orbitz, MD

INDICATION: Myasthenia gravis.

PLASMAPHERESIS NOTE: Today the patient was seen for plasma exchange. He has been tolerating that well. No evidence of hypocalcemic symptoms. Will continue with that today and hopefully will know the results of his antibodies by late afternoon, then I will make a decision whether to continue with that or not.

CPT Code(s): ______________________________

ICD-10-CM Code(s): ______________________________

ICD-9-CM Code(s): ______________________________

Abstracting Questions

1. Does the blood component being exchanged affect the assignment of the apheresis service code? __________

Case 3-3: Catheterization

OPERATIVE REPORT

LOCATION: Inpatient, Hospital

PATIENT: Bob Busch

ATTENDING PHYSICIAN: George Orbitz, MD

PROCEDURE: Tunneled dialysis catheter placement.

INDICATIONS: Plasma exchange for acute crescentic necrotizing glomerulonephritis.

PROCEDURE: After obtaining consent from this 4-year-old patient's parents and localizing the right IJ vein using the Site-Rite machine, his right IJ area was prepped in the usual fashion; 1% lidocaine was used for local anesthesia. The right IJ vein was accessed without difficulty under real-time ultrasound guidance. Guidewire was advanced smoothly. Dilatation was obtained. When dilatation was done, a 16-cm 11.5 French temporary dialysis catheter with curved extension was advanced through the right IJ over the guidewire using the Seldinger technique without difficulty. The catheter was tunneled and was secured to the skin. The patient tolerated the procedure very well without immediate complications. Chest x-ray was ordered.

CPT Code(s): ______________________________

ICD-10-CM Code(s): ______________________________

ICD-9-CM Code(s): ______________________________

Abstracting Questions

1. What was the name of the machine used in this procedure? ______________________________
2. What was the function of the machine in question 1? ______________________________
3. What type of technique was employed in this procedure? ______________________________

Case 3-4: Coronary Artery Bypass Graft

OPERATIVE REPORT

LOCATION: Inpatient, Hospital

PATIENT: A. G. Vanyo

ATTENDING/ADMIT PHYSICIAN: Frank Gaul, MD

SURGEON: James Noonar, MD

PREOPERATIVE DIAGNOSIS: Atherosclerotic heart disease.

POSTOPERATIVE DIAGNOSIS: Atherosclerotic heart disease.

PROCEDURE: Coronary artery bypass graft times two of the left internal mammary artery to the left anterior descending bypass and a single saphenous vein bypass from the aorta to the obtuse marginal branch of the left circumflex.

ANESTHESIA: General.

INDICATION: This 76-year-old male patient with accelerating angina was noted on cardiac catheterization to have high-grade ostial left main coronary disease. He also had a 70% obtuse marginal branch lesion. The left ventricular function was normal.

FINDINGS AT SURGERY: The left anterior descending artery was diffusely diseased throughout and measured 1.5 mm in diameter where it was grafted and was of poor quality. The internal mammary artery was a 2-mm vessel of good quality with excellent flow. The vein was a 6-mm diameter vessel of poor quality, somewhat varicosed, and was used in a reversed fashion. It was not harvested with the endoscopic technique because of the patient's unstable presentation. The obtuse marginal branch was a 2-mm diameter vessel and was of good quality.

PROCEDURE: On May 8 of this year the patient was brought to the operating room and placed in the supine position, and under general intubation anesthesia, the anterior chest, abdomen, and legs were prepped and draped in the usual manner. A segment of greater saphenous vein was harvested from the left thigh and prepared for grafting. The sternum was opened in the usual fashion, and the left internal mammary artery taken down and prepared for grafting. The pericardium was incised sharply, and pericardial well created. The patient was systemically heparinized and placed on single right atrial to aortic cardiopulmonary bypass with a sump in the main pulmonary artery for cardiac decompression. The patient was cooled to 26°C, and on fibrillation, the aortic crossclamp was applied to potassium-rich cold crystalline cardioplegic solution administered through the aortic root with satisfactory cardiac arrest. Subsequent doses were given via the coronary sinus in retrograde fashion and down the vein graft as the anastomosis was completed. The end of the greater saphenous vein was then anastomosed to the proximal portion of the obtuse marginal branch with 7–0 Prolene. The left internal mammary artery was then brought down to the junction of the middle and distal one third of the left anterior descending and anastomosed thereto with 8–0 continuous Prolene. Please note that all grafts were pro patent prior to closure. The aortic crossclamp was removed after 47.6 minutes with spontaneous cardioversion to a normal sinus rhythm. The patient was then warmed to 37°C esophageal temperature and weaned from cardiopulmonary bypass without difficulty after 72 minutes. No inotropes were used. The patient was decannulated, protamine given, and hemostasis achieved. Temporary pacer wires were placed in the right atrium and right ventricle. The chest was drained with two chest tubes and closed in layers in the usual fashion. The leg was closed similarly. Sterile compression dressings were applied, and the patient returned to surgical intensive care unit in satisfactory condition. Sponge count and needle count correct times two.

CPT Code(s): ______________________________

ICD-10-CM Code(s): ______________________________

ICD-9-CM Code(s): ______________________________

Abstracting Questions

1. Was the grafting done with arterial grafts, venous grafts, or both? ______________________________
2. What code range was referenced for assignment of the venous grafting code? ______________________________
3. Was the arterial grafting a single graft or multiple grafts? ______________________________
4. Was the harvesting of the vein graft reported separately? ______________________________
5. Was the cardiopulmonary bypass and cooling reported by the cardiologist? ______________________________

Case 3-5: Intubation

OPERATIVE REPORT

LOCATION: Inpatient, Hospital

PATIENT: Isaac Lock

ATTENDING/ADMIT PHYSICIAN: Frank Gaul, MD

SURGEON: Gregory Dawson, MD

PROCEDURE PERFORMED: Intubation with a #8.5 endotracheal tube and placement on a volume cycle ventilator.

The patient is having acute respiratory failure. He was sedated but is still agitated and combative, and he needs a pacemaker for symptomatic bradycardia. This was an intubation to get the patient under control so they can have an adequate airway while the patient is undergoing a pacemaker placement.

With usual vecuronium and Versed sedation and muscle relaxant, on a one-pass maneuver the patient was intubated with #8.5 endotracheal tube and placed on a volume cycle ventilator without difficulty. We made good capnograph measurement of CO_2, so we knew we were in the airway. A chest x-ray showed good positioning and placement on a volume cycle ventilator. Please see the orders for those settings.

CPT Code(s): ______________________

ICD-10-CM Code(s): ______________________

ICD-9-CM Code(s): ______________________

Abstracting Questions

1. Is the ventilator reported separately? ______________________
2. Is the chest x-ray reported separately by the performing provider? ______________________

Case 3-6: Dressing Change and Oversewing of Tracheostomy

OPERATIVE REPORT

LOCATION: Inpatient, Hospital

PATIENT: Fern Nay

ATTENDING/ADMIT PHYSICIAN: Frank Gaul, MD

SURGEON: Jeff King, MD

PREOPERATIVE DIAGNOSIS: Bleeding from tracheostomy site.

POSTOPERATIVE DIAGNOSIS: Bleeding from tracheostomy site.

PROCEDURE: Dressing change and oversewing of bleeding site of the tracheostomy.

INDICATION: The patient had undergone a tracheostomy 3 days ago. The next day she had been oozing. We have performed a number of changes of Surgicel and silver nitrate, and we were able to get the bleeding to stop that night. Yesterday, although she has never been frankly bleeding, there has been an ooze. We have had to change the dressings about every 4 hours or so; thus, no frank hemorrhage. Minimal to no blood in the tracheostomy on suctions. She just today has started oozing again. I think a lot of this is due to her underlying myeloproliferative disease. We just cannot seem to get the oozing to stop. We therefore did another dressing change under sterile technique and opened up the wound a little bit by removing the lateral sutures to expose this completely.

PROCEDURE: The wound was prepped and draped in the sterile fashion. We removed the lateral skin closure sutures of Prolene. We cleaned out the old Surgicel and old clots. We identified a site on the right side in the soft tissues that seemed to be oozing. This was oversewn with a 4–0 Vicryl. A couple of the small areas were also cauterized. Also, on the left side there was one area that was cauterized. We also infiltrated some of the areas with 1% Xylocaine for local anesthesia. We also sedated her with Versed 2 mg times two doses and 50 mcg of fentanyl. We then just watched the wound for a little bit. It seemed to be staying dry. We packed with Surgicel, Vaseline gauze, and then 4 × 4 silk at the tracheostomy site and reattached the tracheostomy collar. The patient tolerated the procedure well. For the bell alarm, the patient was grounded to her right thigh.

CPT Code(s): ______________________________

ICD-10-CM Code(s): ______________________________

ICD-9-CM Code(s): ______________________________

Abstracting Questions

1. Was the dressing change performed under anesthesia reported separately? ______________
2. Was this procedure a revised tracheostomy or a tracheostoma revision? ______________
3. Is there a secondary diagnosis to report? ______________

Case 3-7: Thoracentesis

OPERATIVE REPORT

LOCATION: Inpatient, Hospital

PATIENT: Dorrie Huot

ATTENDING/ADMIT PHYSICIAN: Frank Gaul, MD

SURGEON: Gary Sanchez, MD

PROCEDURE PERFORMED: Diagnostic thoracentesis, four-quadrant pleural biopsy and pleural drainage with a small-caliber temporary chest tube.

Once the usual scrub was made over the ultrasound mark of the left lateral posterior chest wall, the area was cleansed with Betadine solution and then anesthetized with a total of 20 cc of 1% lidocaine. The cutaneous, subcutaneous, and periosteum of the rib were anesthetized in an area about the size of a 50-cent piece. Once this was accomplished, a small-caliber needle was inserted in the pleural space at the ultrasound mark, and milky white fluid was removed. We had a total of about 50 cc of that fluid for various studies including hematology, chemistry, and bacteriology.

Once that was accomplished, using a small #11 blade, an X incision was made in the cutaneous and subcutaneous tissue, and then a Cope pleural biopsy needle was pushed into position, and the four quadrants were biopsied, carefully avoiding, of course, the noon position. Fragments were sent for pathology. Once this was accomplished, a small-caliber temporary chest tube, i.e., Cook disposable pneumothorax set, was pushed into position. Once it was in position and we were assured we had the same pleural fluid removal site, it was attached to a suction bottle, and 1500 cc of fluid was removed. There were no obvious consequences other than some nausea and vomiting from the patient, but no pain, no shortness of breath. Chest x-ray will be taken post procedure to assure ourselves of a good result, and we will send the fluid we obtained for cytology.

This has the appearance of a chylous effusion. I am sure the patient has some lymph nodes eroded to the thoracic duct, and I will do the various workups to which we are accustomed to make sure we do not overlook anything. Hopefully we will make a diagnosis, and we will have to think about how to control this.

CPT Code(s): ____________________

ICD-10-CM Code(s): ____________________

ICD-9-CM Code(s): ____________________

Abstracting Questions

1. Was the main procedure the thoracentesis or the pleural biopsy? ____________________
2. Was the biopsy open or by means of a needle? ____________________
3. Why does the "X" incision not make this an open procedure? ____________________
4. Is the pleural drainage separately reported? ____________________
5. What is the term that describes the insertion of a chest tube? ____________________.

Case 3-8: Endarterectomy

OPERATIVE REPORT

Report the services of Dr. Sanchez for the following surgical procedure and the EEG monitoring.

LOCATION: Inpatient, Hospital

PATIENT: Jay Hugh

ATTENDING/ADMIT PHYSICIAN: Frank Gaul, MD

SURGEON: Gary Sanchez, MD

PREOPERATIVE DIAGNOSIS: Left carotid stenosis.

POSTOPERATIVE DIAGNOSIS: Left carotid stenosis.

PROCEDURE PERFORMED: Left carotid endarterectomy.

EEG monitoring was utilized throughout the case, and there were no changes at the surgery.

PROCEDURE: Under general anesthesia, the patient's left neck was prepped and draped in the usual manner. An incision was made along the medial border of the sternocleidomastoid. The platysma was incised. Then with sharp dissection we got onto the common carotid artery. I placed the Ligaloop around the common carotid artery, followed the common carotid artery up until I could isolate the internal and external carotid arteries, and placed Ligaloops around the arteries. Having isolated the arteries, I dissected up on the internal carotid artery so that I could have adequate access to the arteriotomy. Having performed this, I placed the Farley-Thompson retractor into the wound. I had good exposure. I then gave the patient 5000 units of heparin IV. I waited 5 minutes, then put the clamps on internal, common, and external carotid arteries, did the arteriotomy, and removed the plaque. This was plaque with clot in it. The artery was very thinned out, but we were able to remove it. I then began suturing of the artery with 5–0 Prolene starting at the distal end, then at the proximal end, producing back bleeding, irritating the inside of the artery with heparinized saline prior to this, and then closing the artery. This reestablished flow up the external first and then up the internal carotid artery. There were small leaks in the suture line. I used 5–0 and 6–0 Prolene to stop them. Circulation having been reestablished, I used some Hemocele on the artery. I placed a Hemovac drain in the wound and closed the wound in layers using 2–0 chromic on the platysma, 2–0 plain in the subcutaneous tissue, and surgical staples on the skin. A dressing was applied. The patient was discharged to the recovery room.

CPT Code(s): ______________________________

ICD-10-CM Code(s): ______________________________

ICD-9-CM Code(s): ______________________________

Abstracting Questions

1. How does the occurrence of a clot in the carotid artery affect the code assignment of this procedure? __________
2. Does the "intraoperative" aspect of the EEG affect code assignment? ______________________________

Case 3-9: Angiogram

Assign the codes for the catheterizations only.

RADIOLOGY REPORT

LOCATION: Inpatient, Hospital

PATIENT: Joy Gigel

ORDERING PHYSICIAN: John Hodgson, MD

ATTENDING/ADMIT PHYSICIAN: Frank Gaul, MD

RADIOLOGIST: Morton Monson, MD

PERSONAL PHYSICIAN: Frank Gaul, MD

EXAMINATION: Carotid/cerebral angiogram.

CLINICAL SYMPTOMS: Intracranial bleed.

CAROTID/CEREBRAL ANGIOGRAM: The patient is a 54-year-old female who was found to have an intracranial bleed. Carotid/cerebral angiogram was requested by Dr. Hodgson, neurosurgery.

APPROACH: Right common femoral artery.

VESSELS INJECTED
1. Proximal thoracic aorta.
2. Right common carotid artery.
3. Right internal carotid artery.
4. Left common carotid artery.
5. Left vertebral artery.

FOLLOW-UP: Dr. Hodgson.
Prior to the start of the study, the procedure was explained to the patient's husband by Dr. Hodgson, including risks, complications, and alternatives. The patient's husband understood and consented to the exam. This study was performed on an emergency basis.

The patient was prepped and draped in the usual sterile fashion. Utilizing single wall technique following administration of local anesthesia (1% lidocaine), a #5 French flush catheter was introduced into the right common femoral artery through a vascular sheath, and the tip was advanced into the proximal thoracic aorta. Contrast was injected, and sequential digital subtraction angiography films were obtained.

The flush catheter was then exchanged for a #4 French Osborne catheter for select evaluation of both common carotid arteries, as well as the right internal carotid artery and the left vertebral artery. Again, contrast was injected, and multiple views of the carotid bifurcations and cerebral vessels were obtained.

On arch injection, there is no significant stenosis at the origin of the great vessels. There is an antegrade flow in both vertebral arteries. Please note that the right vertebral artery is somewhat smaller when compared to the left.

On evaluation of the carotid bifurcations, there is no evidence of narrowing or irregularity.

On evaluation of cerebral vessels, there is no evidence of aneurysm, extravasation, or arteriovenous malformation. Please note that there is marked medial and superior displacement of the vessels in the right middle cerebral artery distribution. There is also midline shift of all the cerebral structures of the left as well as midline shift to the left of the anterior cerebral arteries. These findings are consistent with the patient's intraparenchymal bleed predominantly in the right temporal lobe seen on CT study from an outside institution.

The patient tolerated the procedure well. The puncture site was closed with sutures utilizing the Perclose device. There was no evidence of bleeding, hematoma, or change in peripheral pulses at the termination of the study.

IMPRESSION: Carotid/cerebral angiogram with multiple findings as described above.

Dr. Hodgson was present during this examination.

CPT Code(s): ______________________________

ICD-10-CM Code(s): ______________________________

ICD-9-CM Code(s): ______________________________

Abstracting Questions

1. What CPT Appendix could you reference to understand how to code the procedure performed in the report?

   ____
2. What vessels were evaluated? ______________________________
3. Are right and left HCPCS modifiers appended to the catheter insertion codes? ______________________________
4. Are both the right common carotid and right internal carotid reported? ______________________________
5. Is the left common carotid reported? ______________________________
6. Is the left vertebral artery reported? ______________________________
7. Why does the proximal thoracic aorta not get reported? ______________________________

Case 3-10: Intra-aortic Balloon Pump

OPERATIVE REPORT

LOCATION: Inpatient, Hospital

PATIENT: Barbara Smith

ATTENDING/ADMIT PHYSICIAN: James Noonar, MD

SURGEON: David Barton, MD

INDICATION: Severe left main atherosclerotic heart disease.

DESCRIPTION OF PROCEDURE: The #6 French arterial sheath was exchanged for an intra-aortic balloon pump sheath that was inserted percutaneously. The 40-cc #8 French intra-aortic balloon pump was inserted under fluoroscopic guidance over the guidewire and was advanced to the junction between the aortic arch and the descending thoracic aorta. We pulled the sheath, and the balloon pump was then sutured in place. The patient tolerated the procedure well and suffered no complications. Intra-aortic balloon pumping was started at 1:2 ratio.

CPT Code(s): ______________________________

ICD-10-CM Code(s): ______________________________

ICD-9-CM Code(s): ______________________________

Abstracting Questions

1. What approach was used to insert the device? ______________________________

Chapter 4
Integumentary

Make sure to check evolve learning system for the latest content updates

Case 4-1: Excision, Cheek Lesion

OPERATIVE REPORT

LOCATION: Outpatient, Hospital

PATIENT: Mary Carbono

ATTENDING PHYSICIAN: Gary Sanchez, MD

SURGEON: Gary Sanchez, MD

PREOPERATIVE DIAGNOSIS: Right cheek lesion, unspecified behavior.

POSTOPERATIVE DIAGNOSIS: Right cheek lesion, unspecified behavior.

PROCEDURE PERFORMED: Excision of lesion, right cheek.

ANESTHESIA: General anesthetic by inhalational mask technique.

PROCEDURE: Following informed consent from the patient's mother, the patient was taken to the operating room and placed supine on the operating room table. The appropriate monitoring devices were placed on the patient, and general anesthesia was induced. It was maintained by inhalation mask technique. The right cheek was prepped and draped in a sterile fashion. The lesion, which was about 1.6 cm, somewhat raised, and erythematous, was injected at its base with 0.5 cc of 1% Xylocaine with 1:100,000 epinephrine. A #15-blade scalpel was used to perform a shave excision. No suture was placed. A sterile bandage was applied. The patient tolerated the procedure well. She was allowed to recover from general anesthesia and was transferred to the recovery room in good condition.

Pathology Report Later Indicated: Benign lesion of cheek.

CPT Code(s): ____________________

ICD-10-CM Code(s): ____________________

ICD-9-CM Code(s): ____________________

Abstracting Questions

1. What method was used to excise the lesion? ______
2. Does the pathologic status of the report affect CPT code assignment? ______
3. Does the size and location of the lesion affect CPT code assignment? ______
4. Does the pathologic status of the lesion affect the diagnosis code? ______

Case 4-2: Right Breast Wide Excision

OPERATIVE REPORT

LOCATION: Outpatient, Hospital

PATIENT: Jane Doe

ATTENDING PHYSICIAN: Gary Sanchez, MD

SURGEON: Gary Sanchez, MD

PREOPERATIVE DIAGNOSIS: Mass, right breast.

POSTOPERATIVE DIAGNOSIS: Mass, right breast.

OPERATIVE PROCEDURE: Right breast mass excision.

PROCEDURE: With the patient under general anesthesia, the breast and chest were prepped and draped in a sterile manner. An elliptical incision was made about the palpated mass, including the area around the nipple. This was excised all the way down to the fascia of the breast and then submitted for frozen section. Frozen section revealed a carcinoma of the breast with what appeared to be a good margin all the way around it. We then maintained hemostasis with electrocautery and proceeded to close the breast tissue using 2–0 and 3–0 chromic. The skin was closed using 4–0 Vicryl in a subcuticular manner. Steri-Strips were applied. The patient tolerated the procedure well and was discharged from the operating room in stable condition.

Pathology Report Later Indicated: Primary, malignant neoplasm of the right breast nipple.

CPT Code(s): ______________________________

ICD-10-CM Code(s): ______________________________

ICD-9-CM Code(s): ______________________________

Abstracting Questions

1. Does the pathologic status of the lesion affect CPT code assignment? ______________
2. Does the size of the lesion affect CPT code assignment? ______________
3. Does the pathologic status of the lesion affect the diagnosis code? ______________
4. Does the location of the lesion affect the diagnosis code? ______________
5. Does the gender of the patient affect either code? ______________

Case 4-3: Thenar Flap Coverage

OPERATIVE REPORT

Assign an E code to indicate how this injury occurred in addition to the diagnosis and service codes.

LOCATION: Outpatient, Hospital

PATIENT: Leslie May

ATTENDING PHYSICIAN: Gary Sanchez, MD

SURGEON: Gary Sanchez, MD

PREOPERATIVE DIAGNOSIS: Oblique volar amputation tip, right middle finger, while working on machinery.

POSTOPERATIVE DIAGNOSIS: Oblique volar amputation tip, right middle finger, while working on machinery.

PROCEDURE: Thenar flap coverage, tip, right middle finger.

ANESTHESIA: General.

PROCEDURE: The patient was brought to the operating room, and general anesthesia was induced. Right upper extremity was prepped with Betadine and draped in a sterile fashion. The limb was exsanguinated with a tourniquet inflated to 250 mm Hg for 45 minutes. Using 4× magnification loupes, we debrided the fingertip. It was a volar oblique amputation. However, there was loss of distal phalanx down to about half of the sterile nail matrix. We trimmed the nail plate back to the level of the bone, we debrided the wound, and it was quite clean. We then fabricated a thenar flap using a piece of paper glove as a template. We traced this out on the thenar eminence. We then incised this and elevated the flap with fatty tissue. The radialward digital nerve to the index finger was exposed, and we covered this over with muscle with 4–0 Vicryl suture. We next harvested a split-thickness skin graft from the ulnar aspect of the hand using the Davol dermatome. We then placed this graft in place and sutured it over the defect in the palm with 5–0 Vicryl suture. Tegaderm was then placed over the donor site on the ulnar aspect of the hand.

We then placed the finger down in the palm and then attached the flap with interrupted 5–0 nylon sutures. This covered the defect on the finger nicely. We next applied Xeroform over all wounds and applied wet cotton balls over the graft site to hold it in place, then placed as compression a hand bandage with fluffs, Kerlix, Kling, and plaster splints immobilizing the hand in an intrinsic plus position. The tourniquet was released, and good circulation returned to the hand.

The patient tolerated the procedure well. She went to the recovery room in excellent condition. She will be dismissed as an outpatient today with plans for follow-up back in the office in appropriately 2 weeks.

CPT Code(s): ______________________________

ICD-10-CM Code(s): ______________________________

ICD-9-CM Code(s): ______________________________

Abstracting Questions

1. Was this an adjacent tissue transfer flap? ______
2. Was the CPT code selection based on the recipient or donor site? ______
3. Can the split-thickness skin graft for repair of the donor site be reported separately? ______
4. What HCPCS modifier would be appropriate to append to the CPT code reported for the formation of the pedicle flap? ______
5. Does the way in which the amputation occurred affect the diagnosis code selection? ______
6. If the type of machinery used during the procedure were specified, what other type of diagnosis code would you have reported? ______

Case 4-4: Division and Insert of Flap

OPERATIVE REPORT

The same patient as in Case 4-3 is returned to the operating room after previously having a flap applied to the middle right fingertip, which was traumatically amputated. This is a staged procedure within the postoperative period, and often after the procedure any unused portions of the flap or previous skin grafts are removed and/or returned to anatomic sites.

LOCATION: Outpatient, Hospital

PATIENT: Leslie May

ATTENDING PHYSICIAN: Gary Sanchez, MD

SURGEON: Gary Sanchez, MD

PREOPERATIVE DIAGNOSIS: Status post thenar flap, right middle fingertip due to oblique volar amputation.

POSTOPERATIVE DIAGNOSIS: Status post thenar flap, right middle fingertip due to oblique volar amputation.

PROCEDURE PERFORMED: Division and insetting of thenar flap, right middle finger and palm.

ANESTHESIA: General.

PROCEDURE: The patient was brought to the operating room, and general anesthesia was induced. The right upper extremity was removed from the bandages. We prepped it with Betadine and draped it in a sterile fashion. We then exsanguinated the limb, and a tourniquet was inflated to 250 mm Hg for 30 minutes. We then divided the flap. Attention was first directed to the thenar eminence. There was no sign of infection. The sutures were removed, and we lightly debrided some of the scarring. We then inset the flap and sutured this with interrupted 5–0 nylon suture. We then inspected the fingertip. All sutures were removed. The flap was viable. There was no sign of infection at the flap proximally. We inset the flap proximally and set this in with interrupted 5–0 nylon suture. The nail plate had elevated off the nailbed, and we therefore cleansed dried blood from underneath the nailbed. There was no sign of infection. We irrigated this with sterile saline. We then applied Xeroform over all wounds, and we placed a compression bandage across the palm and also TubeGauz bandage on the finger. Tourniquet was released, and good circulation returned to the hand.

The patient will be dismissed as an outpatient today with plans for follow-up back in the office in 7-10 days.

DISCHARGE MEDICATIONS: Darvocet-N 100, 30 tablets.

CPT Code(s): ______________________________

ICD-10-CM Code(s): ______________________________

ICD-9-CM Code(s): ______________________________

Abstracting Questions

1. Does the fact that there was a flap affect code assignment? ______________________
2. What CPT modifier is required to correctly report this staged procedure? ______________________

Case 4-5: Laceration Repair

OPERATIVE REPORT

Assign an E code to indicate how the injury occurred.

LOCATION: Outpatient, Hospital

PATIENT: Rod Seim

ATTENDING PHYSICIAN: Gary Sanchez, MD

SURGEON: Gary Sanchez, MD

PREOPERATIVE DIAGNOSIS: Multiple simple lacerations, right middle finger due to arrow.

POSTOPERATIVE DIAGNOSIS: Multiple simple lacerations, right middle finger due to arrow.

PROCEDURE PERFORMED: Simple closure of lacerations to right middle finger.

ANESTHESIA: Ring block.

PROCEDURE: Ring block anesthesia was achieved with 1% Xylocaine without epinephrine. Once the ring block was successful, the patient was taken to the scrub sink and the finger gently scrubbed and thoroughly irrigated with water. Once the finger was cleansed, repair was performed. The patient had a small nick (1 cm) in the lateral band. This was tacked together with one 4–0 nylon suture. There was noted to be no dirt on the tendon after irrigating the finger. To minimize the risk for infection, it was elected to just loosely close this. The 5-cm, J-shaped wound was then closed with four 4–0 nylon sutures just to approximate the skin. Some fat at the edge of the volar wound was debrided with scissors, and some abrasion of the epidermis was also debrided with scissors. The volar wound was then closed with two 4–0 nylon sutures. Dressing and a TubeGauz dressing were then applied. The patient tolerated this well.

CPT Code(s): ______________________________

ICD-10-CM Code(s): ______________________________

ICD-9-CM Code(s): ______________________________

Abstracting Questions

1. What type of repair was performed (simple, intermediate, complex)? ______________
2. Does the location on the body of the repair affect the choice of the CPT code assignment? ______________
3. Does the size of the repair affect the choice of CPT code? ______________
4. The 7th character on the ICD-10-CM code indicates this was a/an ______________ encounter.
5. Does the repair to the nick in the tendon affect the diagnosis coding? ______________

Case 4-6: Massive Debridement

OPERATIVE REPORT

LOCATION: Inpatient, Hospital

PATIENT: Pam Tieg

ATTENDING PHYSICIAN: Leslie Alanda, MD

SURGEON: Gary Sanchez, MD

PREOPERATIVE DIAGNOSES
1. Massive abdominal wound.
2. Status post multiple small-bowel fistula repair.

POSTOPERATIVE DIAGNOSES
1. Massive abdominal wound.
2. Status post multiple small-bowel fistula repair.

SURGICAL FINDINGS: There was a 28 × 50-cm open wound in the abdomen extending predominantly to the right over past the midline on the left with a more inferior extension near the inguinal ligament. The primary areas of concern were pockets that were at least 8 to 10 cm in diameter in their total dimensions that had undermined in the retroperitoneal space behind the bowel. This contained malodorous fat necrosis and other necrotic tissue, and the odor smelled like Gram-negative organisms. We noted that the bowel was anterior in this space and probably came down on the psoas muscle posteriorly on the right side. Also, there were various areas of fat necrosis overlying the superficial aspect of the wound and fat necrosis along the edges of the wound that was quite malodorous. Multiple cultures and sensitivities were obtained, particularly of the area around the ileostomy site, the large area of fat necrosis in the left side of the abdomen, and the two undermined retroperitoneal areas. There was some extrusion of the mesh with the surrounding coagulative necrosis superiorly.

SURGICAL PROCEDURE: Massive debridement of open abdominal wound and status post multiple enterotomy repairs, small bowel.

ANESTHESIA: General, administered through tracheostomy tube.

ESTIMATED BLOOD LOSS: Approximately 50 cc.

ADDENDUM: Dr. White was called to observe the wound at his request and advised us regarding the dissection retroperitoneally in the proximity of the bowel in the area.

PROCEDURE: The abdomen was prepped as well as possible considering the conditions with Betadine scrub and solution and draped in a routine sterile fashion. A major 3-cm area of fat necrosis was initially debrided, and I debrided multiple sites of fat necrosis over the exposed surface of the wound, and then along the marginal surface there were multiple sites that were malodorous. Culture and sensitivity were obtained of the original fat necrosis area, the area around the ileostomy, and the more malodorous areas along the skin edges. We then, on the right side, lifted up the abdominal contents and dissected behind this, encountering foul-smelling, anaerobic-smelling collection of tissue, which probably consisted of old blood clot and fat necrosis. This was gently curetted out without entering the bowel. The bowel was in immediate proximity. We came down on what appeared to be the psoas area, which apparently connected with this pocket on the right side. We packed the right side with metronidazole-soaked Kerlix roll and vaginal packing, then also did the same on the left side. We covered the areas of the wound that were most accessible with fine mesh gauze soaked in metronidazole. ABD pads were then applied. The patient tolerated the procedure well and left the area in good condition.

CPT Code(s): ______

ICD-10-CM Code(s): ______

ICD-9-CM Code(s): ______

Abstracting Questions

1. Was debridement superficial, deep, or both? ______
2. Was the skin debridement code selection affected by the infection? ______
3. Does the skin debridement code include the retroperitoneal exploration? ______
4. Was there a CPT code for re-exploration of a recent abdominal surgery site? ______
5. Why would code 11008 not be reported? ______
6. Were there different diagnosis codes required to report the necrotic status of abdominal fat, skin, and retroperitoneum? ______

Case 4-7: Minimal Debridement

OPERATIVE REPORT

The patient is returned to the operating room during the postoperative period of the first procedure reported in Case 4-6.

LOCATION: Inpatient, Hospital

PATIENT: Pam Tieg

ATTENDING PHYSICIAN: Leslie Alanda, MD

SURGEON: Gary Sanchez, MD

PREOPERATIVE DIAGNOSES
1. Massive abdominal wound with multiple sites of fat necrosis and retroperitoneal tissue necrosis, predominantly fat.
2. Draining sinus, anterior abdominal wall.

POSTOPERATIVE DIAGNOSES
1. Massive abdominal wound with multiple sites of fat necrosis and retroperitoneal tissue necrosis, predominantly fat.
2. Draining sinus, anterior abdominal wall.

SURGICAL FINDINGS: There are about 10 sites of fat necrosis scattered throughout the anterior abdominal wall, but the posterior aspect of the wound (i.e., in the retroperitoneal space that is obliterated by the overhang of bowel) appeared to be clean as far as we could tell, and certainly there was no odor.

SURGICAL PROCEDURE
1. Minimal debridement of anterior abdominal wall wound.
2. Collection of specimen for amylase.

ANESTHESIA: General endotracheal.

PROCEDURE: The patient's abdomen was prepped with Betadine scrub and solution and draped in the routine sterile fashion. Multiple sites of fat necrosis were debrided, and one area of protrusion of the mesh was debrided. There was some clear fluid leaking from a sinus in the anterior abdominal wall, and we collected 2 cc of fluid from this and submitted it for amylase. The wound was then repacked with Kerlix-soaked dressings using 0.5% metronidazole, and fine mesh gauze was applied to the anterior abdominal wound. The patient seemed to tolerate the procedure well and left the area in good condition. We additionally did spray Hemaseel into a pocket in the retroperitoneal area where there was some bleeding that did not respond to cautery, and it was thought that this was more the nature of generalized oozing, and therefore the Hemaseel and packing were used for control.

CPT Code(s): ______________________________

ICD-10-CM Code(s): ______________________________

ICD-9-CM Code(s): ______________________________

Abstracting Questions

See Case 4-6

1. Was the retroperitoneum re-explored? ____________________

2. Does the return to the operating room require a modifier appended to the surgical procedure code? __________

Case 4-8: Amputation

Assign an external cause/E code to indicate how the injury occurred.

OPERATIVE REPORT

LOCATION: Outpatient, Hospital

PATIENT: Ray Darwin

PRIMARY CARE PHYSICIAN: Eugene Hightower, MD

SURGEON: Gary Sanchez, MD

PREOPERATIVE DIAGNOSIS: Volar V-Y advancement of the flap, right middle finger.

POSTOPERATIVE DIAGNOSIS: Volar V-Y advancement of the flap, right middle finger.

PROCEDURE PERFORMED: Transverse amputation of the tip of right middle finger.

ANESTHESIA: 0.5% Marcaine local metacarpal block.

PREOPERATIVE NOTE: The patient did sustain an injury yesterday when he cut his dominant right middle fingertip between a dock and a boat as a wave caught the boat at the lake. He was seen at the local emergency room and was given a tetanus booster, and the wound was dressed. He has been scheduled for V-Y advancement flap to the finger today. He is originally from Manytown and will be having follow-up care from his family physician, Dr. Hightower.

After full discussion with the patient, he elects to proceed with this skin flap today.

PROCEDURE: The patient was brought to the operating room, and a metacarpal block was induced with 10 cc of 0.5% Marcaine. The dressings were removed from the right middle finger, and the right upper extremity was prepped with Betadine and draped in a sterile fashion. A digital tourniquet was applied to the finger for approximately 25 minutes. With 4× magnification loupes, we debrided the finger. This was an amputation through the distal end of the sterile nail matrix. About two thirds of the sterile nail matrix and the entire germinal matrix were still present, and the nail plate was absent. Most of the volar pad was still intact. There was about 3 to 4 mm of distal tuft of the distal phalanx that was absent. However, the wound was extremely clean. We lightly debrided it and removed blood clots. We thoroughly irrigated with sterile saline. We then fabricated a volar V-Y advancement flap back to the distal interphalangeal joint flexor crease. We then moved this flap distalward and advanced it about 5 to 6 mm. We then sutured this directly to the nailbed with interrupted 5–0 Vicryl sutures and closed this up along its margins with interrupted 5–0 nylon sutures. The appearance was excellent. We then placed Xeroform into the nailbed proximally to prevent adhesions. We then removed the digital tourniquet, and excellent circulation returned to the fingertip, including vascular blood in the graft. We then applied Xeroform over the wounds with light gauze dressings, TubeGauz, and light Coban. The patient tolerated the procedure well. He will be dismissed as an outpatient today. He will complete his fishing trip and return to Manytown in 2 or 3 days, and he will follow up with his home physician, Dr. Hightower. *(Note that Dr. Sanchez provided only the surgical service.)* Patient has been placed on Keflex 500 mg p.o. q.i.d. for 5 days. We also gave him a prescription for Lorcet, 30 tablets.

CPT Code(s): ______

ICD-10-CM Code(s): ______

ICD-9-CM Code(s): ______

Abstracting Questions

1. Was the skin repair a free flap or an adjacent tissue transfer? ______
2. What modifier is required to indicate that only the intraoperative portion of the service was provided?

   ______
3. What other modifier would be appropriate? ______
4. Which modifier is reported first? ______

Case 4-9: Nevus Excision

OPERATIVE REPORT

One week prior to this report, Dr. Erickson, plastic surgeon, removed a portion of a nevus from the right arm of Leonardo Zapata. Dr. Erickson believed that a further excision was necessary but wanted another opinion. Mr. Zapata was referred to Dr. Matalo to obtain his opinion on the further excision (staged procedure). Dr. Matalo recommended further excision, and today Dr. Erickson performed the other surgery. The follow-up for the first procedure was 10 days.

LOCATION: Outpatient, Hospital

PATIENT: Leonardo Zapata

PRIMARY CARE PHYSICIAN: Ronald Green, MD

SURGEON: Mark Erickson, MD

INDICATION: This patient had a 1-cm lesion excised from the right arm approximately 1 week ago. There was a question as to whether or not this was a Spitz nevus versus melanoma, and this was referred to Dr. Matalo at the New York Clinic for a second opinion. His opinion was that this was a Spitz nevus, and further conservative excision was recommended if that had not already been done. Since we only took a 5-mm margin, we are going to take about another 1 cm or so off around the previously excised area.

PREOPERATIVE DIAGNOSIS: Spitz nevus, right arm.

POSTOPERATIVE DIAGNOSIS: Spitz nevus, right arm.

SURGICAL FINDINGS: A healed incision of the right arm 2 cm in diameter.

ANESTHESIA: Six cc of 1% Xylocaine with 1:100,000 epinephrine.

PROCEDURE: The arm was prepped with Betadine solution and draped in the routine sterile fashion. The lesion was anesthetized and excised elliptically. Bleeders were electrocoagulated, and the wound was closed with interrupted subcuticular 3–0 Monocryl sutures and two twists of 4–0 Prolene. Half-inch Steri-Strips were applied. The patient tolerated the procedure well and left the area in good condition. He will use the sling that he used with his previous incision.

Pathology Report Later Indicated: Nevus, right arm, re-excision. Skin showing biopsy site with fibrosis, granulation tissue, and suture.

CPT Code(s): ____________________

ICD-10-CM Code(s): ____________________

ICD-9-CM Code(s): ____________________

Abstracting Questions

1. Is a modifier required to indicate the patient is in the global period from a previous procedure? ______________
2. What modifier reports a more extensive procedure than the initial procedure performed during the global period of a previous procedure? ______________
3. What was the excised diameter of the initial excision? ______________
4. What is the excised diameter for the re-operation? ______________

Chapter 5

Emergency Medicine

Make sure to check evolve learning system for the latest content updates

Case 5-1: Forearm Abrasion and Swelling

Assign external cause codes/E codes to indicate how the injury occurred and the place of occurrence. Dr. Sutton is an employee of the hospital.

LOCATION: Outpatient, Hospital

PATIENT: Noel Jackson

PRIMARY CARE PHYSICIAN: Ronald Green, MD

ED PHYSICIAN: Paul Sutton, MD

SUBJECTIVE: The patient is an 8-year-old male who presents to the emergency department with complaints of right forearm abrasion and swelling. He was checked into the boards while playing ice hockey at school. He states he could move the wrist and elbow well. He denies any other injuries.

EXAMINATION: Shows an 8-year-old in no acute distress. He has obvious swelling over the dorsal medial aspect of the forearm. He has an abrasion across there as well. He has excellent range of motion at the wrist and hand as well as the elbow. I put pretty good pressure distally and proximally to the abrasion, and it does not seem to have much tenderness. X-rays were taken, and no fractures were appreciated.

ASSESSMENT: Right forearm abrasion and contusion.

PLAN: Ice and antibiotic ointment. Follow up if not improving.

CPT Code(s): ______________________________

ICD-10-CM Code(s): ______________________________

ICD-9-CM Code(s): ______________________________

Abstracting Questions

1. Does the location of service affect the code range for this service? ___________________
2. How many of the three key components must be met/exceeded to report the CPT code level?

   ____
3. What level of history was documented? ___________________
4. What level of examination was documented? ___________________
5. What level of medical decision making was documented? ___________________
6. How many external cause codes/E codes are required to report this incident? ___________________

Case 5-2: Vomiting

Dr. Sutton is an employee of the hospital.

LOCATION: Outpatient, Hospital

PATIENT: Penny Karlin

PRIMARY CARE PHYSICIAN: Ronald Green, MD

ED PHYSICIAN: Paul Sutton, MD

SUBJECTIVE: This is a 50-year-old female who is presenting to the emergency department today with a complaint of vomiting.

HISTORY OF PRESENT ILLNESS: This patient has quite significant recent medical history; recently diagnosed with grade IV esophageal cancer. She has been to the Lato Clinic and evaluated there, as well as in Los Angeles with endoscopy, and eventually to the Lato Clinic for further workup. With her workup there they found that she had quite extensive cancer with metastatic disease to the bones as well as to the stomach and thought that palliative oncologic treatment was all that could be offered and she should return to the area for this. She is scheduled to have a central line placed tomorrow and also considerations to nutritional needs. She stated that over the past several days she has had some fundraisers and some events for her and she really wanted to attend even though she was not able to keep foods and fluids down. She has been taking only small sips at a time. It seems like her ability to swallow is getting quite impaired, and as a result she cannot swallow her pain pill, so she is having severe pain in her back, hip, and abdomen. She has had increasing fatigue, has vomited several times, and just is not doing well and comes in for this at this time.

PAST MEDICAL HISTORY: Remarkable for esophageal cancer grade IV adenocarcinoma, noted with pelvic mets.

MEDICATIONS: Oxycodone and promethazine.

ALLERGIES: NKA, other than latex.

SOCIAL HISTORY: No smoking or alcohol.

REVIEW OF SYSTEMS: Negative for fever or chills. No shortness of breath. No headache. Patient's got nausea and abdominal and lower chest pain as positives on her review of systems.

On admission to the'emergency department today, the patient's vital signs show a temperature of 36.8, pulse of 99, respiratory rate at 18, and blood pressure 132/84. General: This is a 50-year-old female who is awake, alert, and cooperative. HEENT: Head is normocephalic and atraumatic. Pupils are reactive to light. Conjunctivae clear. Nares patent. TMs are clear. Mouth reveals a somewhat dry oropharynx with some chapping of the lips, which appear parched. Neck is supple. Trachea is midline. Examination of lungs reveals clear breath sounds. Cardiovascular: S1 and S2 without murmur, click, or rub. Abdomen is soft. There is mild tenderness to palpation in the epigastric region. No mass, guarding, or rigidity. Extremities are without deformity or edema. Skin exam shows no rash. Cranial nerves 2 through 12 grossly intact. No gross motor or sensory deficits noted at this time.

SUMMARY OF EMERGENCY DEPARTMENT COURSE: The patient is seen and evaluated for the above-mentioned complaint. Orthostatic blood pressures were obtained: lying 112/87 with a pulse of 78, sitting 108/74 with a pulse of 98, and standing 102/80 with a pulse of 116. So she had quite an increase in her heart rate with standing, which I believe is significant. I did start an IV here in the department with normal saline; I gave her a liter of normal saline and 4 mg of morphine for her pain, which did help her pain significantly. It came down from an 8 to a 3. Checked some blood counts and metabolic panel as well as giving her some Phenergan for nausea, and this did help take away the nausea. Her CBC shows a hemoglobin level of 9.1, white count is okay, and her electrolytes are normal. So I think she is on the cusp of dehydration; certainly some anemia present here. I spoke with Dr. Green, who is covering for Dr. White, the patient's oncologist here, and he agreed to come in and evaluate the patient and did admit the patient to his service for further evaluation and treatment.

ASSESSMENT
1. Acute nausea and vomiting and dehydration.
2. Adenocarcinoma of the esophagus with metastatic disease.

PLAN: As above, the patient will be admitted for further evaluation and treatment per Dr. Green, certainly to control her pain, and it looks to me that the patient is going to have to change her pain regimen from oral to either parenteral or transdermal delivery system. She is going to have a line placed tomorrow, and further evaluation and treatment will be based on Dr. Green's plan for the patient. These plans as mentioned above were reviewed with the patient, who was in agreement. She will be admitted in fair condition with poor prognosis.

CPT Code(s): ______________________________

ICD-10-CM Code(s): ______________________________

ICD-9-CM Code(s): ______________________________

Abstracting Questions

1. What level of history was documented? ______________________________
2. What level of examination was documented? ______________________________
3. What level of medical decision making was documented? ______________________________
4. This case began in the emergency department, but what was the ultimate disposition of this patient?

   ____
5. Why is a neoplasm code not the first-listed diagnosis? ______________________________

Case 5-3: Gastroesophageal Reflux Disease

EMERGENCY AND OUTPATIENT RECORD

LOCATION: Outpatient, Hospital

PATIENT: Maxwell Southgate

PRIMARY CARE PHYSICIAN: Ronald Green, MD

ED PHYSICIAN: Paul Sutton, MD

SUBJECTIVE: This is a 66-year-old white male with history of gastroesophageal reflux disease, coronary artery disease, dyslipidemia, and hypertension. He has a pacemaker in place. His medication regimen includes Altace, Ativan, calcium, Coumadin, Lipitor, lutein, multivitamins, Nexium p.r.n., Tylenol, and vitamin E. He has allergies to codeine. He presents to the emergency room. He was brought in by ambulance with a history of fever, nausea, and vomiting off and on for the past week, significantly worsening in the past 24 hours.

REVIEW OF SYSTEMS: Constitutional: He has fevers, as outlined above. Gastrointestinal: No nausea or vomiting. He has had some loose stools. Genitourinary: He describes some urgency, frequency, and some dysuria as well. Respiratory: He has had a slight cough. Feels slightly short of breath. Cardiovascular: No chest pain or peripheral edema.

OBJECTIVE: His temperature is 38.1. Pulse 100 and regular. Respirations 18. O_2 saturation 95% on room air. Blood pressure 143/60. HEENT: He does have dry mucous membranes. Neck: There is no thyromegaly, adenopathy, or venous distention. Heart: S1 and S2. No S3 or S4. Rhythm is regular. Lungs: He has a slight crackle to both bases. Clears slightly with cough. Suspect bronchovesicular sound at the right base. Abdomen: Bowel sounds present and active. No organomegaly. No masses or hernias noted. Some mild diffuse tenderness. No localizing tenderness. No guarding, rebound, or percussion tenderness.

EXTREMITIES: Negative for significant cyanosis or edema.

Chest x-ray shows question of slight strandy infiltrate and change in the right base. Slight bumping of the left costophrenic angle. There is no significant congestive change.

LABORATORY STUDIES: Laboratory studies included a basic metabolic panel with a BUN elevated at 33. Creatinine 1.8. His electrolytes are within normal limits except for calcium low at 7.8. Glucose is 121 nonfasting. PT at 35.8 and INR 9.6, significantly elevated. Complete blood count: White count of 10,170. Normal differential. Hemoglobin of 11.7. Hematocrit 35.8, normal. Normal platelet count. We have ordered two blood cultures. IV and normal saline is administered, 1 liter. He is given 12.5 mg of IV Phenergan. He did have an emesis while in the emergency department. We have also ordered a urinalysis.

ASSESSMENT
1. Febrile illness.
2. Nausea and vomiting and dehydration.
3. Significant elevated PT/INR.

PLAN: Dr. Green, patient's personal physician, was notified and discussed the case. He arrived to evaluate and assume care. The patient was admitted under Dr. Green's service.

CPT Code(s): ______________________________

ICD-10-CM Code(s): ______________________________

ICD-9-CM Code(s): ______________________________

Abstracting Questions

1. What does PT stated in the report refer to? ______________________________
2. What does PT measure? ______________________________

Case 5-4: Headache

EMERGENCY ROOM VISIT

LOCATION: Outpatient, Hospital

PATIENT: Esther Ertel

PRIMARY CARE PHYSICIAN: Wallace Brown, MD

ED PHYSICIAN: Paul Sutton, MD

CHIEF COMPLAINT: Headache.

SUBJECTIVE: A pleasant 32-year-old female presents to the emergency room complaining of severe headache. She was seen apparently in Anytown within the past week with complaint. She has had a headache for the last couple of weeks. It started 2 weeks ago Sunday and came on "all of a sudden." There was no trauma. The patient was hospitalized in Anytown and 5 to 7 days later was given some meperidine and was empirically treated with antibiotics. The headache was significantly improved but not completely gone. Apparently CT was read as normal. She does complain of some nausea. Says the headaches again have gotten worse. No real photophobia. Has some blurry vision in the left eye. Dr. Brown called us today from Anytown concerned about her severe headache and dilated left pupil that started today. She presents to the emergency room for further evaluation. She says her neck is a little bit stiff. Denies any fever. There are no associated symptoms or modifying factors.

For printed past medical history, family history, social history, and review of systems, please see my resident's note.

PHYSICAL EXAMINATION: Vital signs are stable. She is completely alert. HEENT is grossly benign other than marked dilated left pupil of 7 mm. No gross papilledema is noted. Extraocular muscles are full. Cranial nerves are otherwise intact. Lungs are clear. Heart without murmur. Grip strength is equal. Neurologic is nonfocal. Again, she is completely alert. She was previously given some DHE, meperidine, and Toradol in Anytown.

We did obtain a CT scan of the head and discussed the results with Dr. Brown. Patient indeed does have a subarachnoid hemorrhage. He said she does have some early hydrocephalus.

ASSESSMENT: Subarachnoid hemorrhage.

PLAN: She was given 5 mg of IV morphine. I did discuss the patient with Dr. Green of critical care as well as Dr. Pleasant in neurosurgery. They both agree to assume care, and Dr. Green will be seeing the patient up in the intensive care unit. Had a long discussion with the patient, her husband, and son. Their questions were answered to the best of my ability.

CPT Code(s): ______________________________

ICD-10-CM Code(s): ______________________________

ICD-9-CM Code(s): ______________________________

Abstracting Questions

1. This visit began in the emergency department, but what was the ultimate disposition of the patient?

   ____

2. Why would you not report the headache as a diagnosis? ______________________

Case 5-5: Closed Head Injury

Assign external cause codes/E codes to indicate how the injury occurred and the place of occurrence. Dr. Sutton is an employee of the hospital.

LOCATION: Outpatient, Hospital

PATIENT: Lance Wilson

PRIMARY CARE PHYSICIAN: Ronald Green, MD

ED PHYSICIAN: Paul Sutton, MD

HISTORY OF PRESENT ILLNESS: This 3-year-old male was at the grocery store with his mom when he fell out of the cart and landed on his head. He immediately started crying and was initially inconsolable, but then after crying himself out he had a somewhat dazed look on his face that lasted briefly (10 minutes), but mom got very concerned and wanted to bring him in. She brought him home, and dad accompanies mom for the child's evaluation. Mom states the child has been normal, but she is still concerned. Since dad has seen him, the child has been completely appropriate, awake, alert, and acting himself. It has been 1 hour to 1 hour 15 minutes since the incident occurred, but they came in with this complaint. No other abnormalities or complaints noted at this time.

PAST MEDICAL HISTORY: Remarkable for ear infections in the past. He does have a PE tube on the right.

MEDICATIONS: None.

ALLERGIES: NKA.

SOCIAL HISTORY: He lives with his mom and dad.

REVIEW OF SYSTEMS: Negative for loss of consciousness. The patient has not been complaining of a headache. He has been acting appropriately. No vomiting.

Vital signs in the ED show his temperature 35.8, pulse 120, respiratory rate 20. General: This is a well-hydrated and well-nourished–appearing 3-year-old male who is awake and alert looking about the room and interactive with his environment. He is playing with his mom and dad. His head is normocephalic. He has a small contusion on his forehead that is minimally swollen. His pupils are reactive to light. EOMs are intact. Nares are patent. Tympanic membranes are clear. Tubes in the right ear are well placed. Oropharynx is clear. Neck is supple. Trachea is midline. Lungs are clear. Heart is regular. Abdomen soft. Extremities without deformity or edema. Skin examination shows no rash.

SUMMARY OF EMERGENCY DEPARTMENT COURSE: The patient is seen and evaluated with the above-mentioned complaint. I did observe the child here with a full physical examination. He is walking, talking, playful, and acting appropriately. This is about an hour and a half after the incident. Skull films were obtained and were negative. I do think that the child, because of his appropriate behavior and absence of skull fracture and minimal swelling at this time, can follow up with his physician tomorrow for recheck and be sent home with head injury instructions. They can wake the child up every 4 hours and bring him back if he is worse. I think this is a very reasonable approach for this patient given his circumstances. I reviewed this information with his mom and dad. They are in agreement with our treatment plan. It is understood that if the child were to change his behavior, he should be brought back in for re-evaluation; otherwise, he can follow up with his pediatrician in the morning.

ASSESSMENT: Acute closed head injury, grade I concussion.

PLAN: As above. Discharge to home. Follow up with his pediatrician tomorrow. Tylenol or Motrin as needed; return if any abnormal behavior, vomiting; and please read head injury instructions.

CPT Code(s): ______________________________

ICD-10-CM Code(s): ______________________________

ICD-9-CM Code(s): ______________________________

Abstracting Questions

1. Why did the physician direct the parents to wake the child every 4 hours? ______________________________
2. What are the two most prominent symptoms that indicated this was a grade I concussion? ____________________

Case 5-6: Sore Throat, Earache, and Sore Chest

Dr. Sutton is an employee of the hospital.

LOCATION: Outpatient, Hospital

PATIENT: George Brown

PRIMARY CARE PHYSICIAN: Frank Gaul, MD

ED PHYSICIAN: Paul Sutton, MD

SUBJECTIVE: This is a 25-year-old male presenting to the ED today with complaint of sore throat, earache, and sore chest, as well as a cough.

HISTORY OF PRESENT ILLNESS: Symptoms present for the past 4–5 days. He states it started with some soreness in his chest. He has been having a cough, and now he has developed an earache over the last 24 hours, and this is the most significant problem at this time. He also states an irritation and soreness to the throat. No significant fevers. He has had mild chills; no nausea, vomiting, or diarrhea and presents for evaluation.

PAST MEDICAL HISTORY: Remarkable for no chronic medical conditions, no medications or allergies.

MEDICATIONS: None.

ALLERGIES: NKA.

SOCIAL HISTORY: Nonsmoker.

REVIEW OF SYSTEMS: Negative for fevers; no vomiting or nausea. Positive for sore throat, muscle aches, cough, chest soreness, and earache. Vital signs in the department show his temperature 36.4, pulse 69, respiratory rate 16, blood pressure 119/81, sat is 99% on room air.

General Exam: This is an awake, alert, well-hydrated, well-nourished–appearing 25-year-old male who is alert, oriented, and cooperative. HEENT: Head normocephalic and atraumatic. Pupils are reactive to light. Conjunctivae are clear. Nares are patent. Mouth reveals a moist oropharynx with mild erythema in the posterior pharynx. Left TM is erythematous and retracted. Neck is supple, and no significant anterior adenopathy. Trachea is midline. Lungs are clear. Heart is regular. Abdomen is soft and nontender, nondistended; bowel sounds are active. Extremities show no evidence of deformity or edema. Skin exam shows no rash.

The patient presents with symptoms of influenza. I did do a screen that was negative. In light of this, will treat him for his otitis media. I am not going to do a strep screen on him; it does not look characteristic for strep. Will treat him with Vantin 200 mg p.o. q.d. for a week. A prescription was given. He was also given a dose here in the department. Auralgan was placed in his left ear, which afforded him significant improvement in his pain, and he was very pleased with this.

DISCHARGE DIAGNOSES
1. Acute left otitis media.
2. Viral upper respiratory infection.

CPT Code(s): ______________________________

ICD-10-CM Code(s): ______________________________

ICD-9-CM Code(s): ______________________________

Abstracting Questions

1. Would the discharge diagnoses be the same as the presenting problems? ______________
2. What does the abbreviation NKA stand for? ______________

Case 5-7: Thigh Redness

Dr. Sutton is an employee of the hospital.

LOCATION: Outpatient, Hospital

PATIENT: Shawn Bailey

ED PHYSICIAN: Paul Sutton, MD

SUBJECTIVE: This 20-year-old male presents to the ED today with a complaint of redness of the left thigh. Patient states his symptoms started yesterday with a pimple-like boil located in the medial aspect of the left thigh. He stated this area was slightly painful and red, and since that time he has tried to pop and squeeze it, but really did not get any pus out of the lesion. Since yesterday it has become much larger in size, and now it is greater than the size of the palm and seems to be spreading. He has some redness. He notes some swelling in his groin, which he thinks is a tender lymph node. He states that he was having some discomfort with his leg. He states that he had felt warm, but had not had a measured temp. He has taken aspirin, which helped both the pain and his feeling of a fever. He has not taken anything else for this. He comes in for evaluation at this time. He does not have any known history of diabetes.

PAST MEDICAL HISTORY: No pertinent medical problems. No known history of diabetes. Patient takes no medications, has no allergies.

SOCIAL HISTORY: He is a nonsmoker and uses no alcohol.

REVIEW OF SYSTEMS: Negative for fever, chills, vomiting, or frequent urination.

EXAMINATION: Vital signs in the emergency department show his temperature at 95°F, pulse steady with respiratory rate of 16, blood pressure 125/75. General exam shows a well-nourished 20-year-old male who is awake, alert, and oriented. Heart is regular. Lungs are clear. Focused exam of the right leg shows inguinal lymphadenopathy, which is very minimal, but tender. There is no redness streaking up the leg, but he does have a palm-sized area of cellulitis that is outlined in tandem with the warmth and redness. The center is scabbed, which is only about 0.5 cm in size. There is a small amount of induration, but no fluctuance in this area. Distal extremities are unremarkable, and he has no edema. Patient generally looks nontoxic. He is cooperative and pleasant at this time.

SUMMARY OF EMERGENCY DEPARTMENT COURSE: Patient was seen and evaluated with the above-mentioned chief complaint. He was given 800 mg of p.o. Motrin and 2 grams of Ancef, along with a script for medications at home. I want him to follow up tomorrow, or sooner if the redness seems to grow beyond the point demarcated for him. Patient is well aware of the instructions and is agreeable to follow these. I am going to give him the name of a doctor for follow-up tomorrow as well.

ASSESSMENT: Acute cellulitis, right thigh.

PLAN: Patient did receive Ancef 2 grams here. I am going to have him start regularly in the morning with Keflex 500 q.i.d. for 7 days. He can take Motrin 600 mg every 6 hours for pain and discomfort, and the Motrin here did help, so I think this will be good for that aspect of his care. I would like to have him follow up with physician who was assigned to him on discharge for re-evaluation within 24 hours.

CPT Code(s): ______

ICD-10-CM Code(s): ______

ICD-9-CM Code(s): ______

Abstracting Questions

1. Why was modifier -LT not added to the CPT code for this service? ______
2. What was the definition of "medial aspect" as used in this report? ______

Case 5-8: Patellar Dislocation

Assign external cause codes/E codes to indicate how the injury occurred and the place of occurrence. Dr. Sutton is an employee of the hospital.

LOCATION: Outpatient, Hospital

PATIENT: Tiffany Haney

PRIMARY CARE PHYSICIAN: Ronald Green, MD

ED PHYSICIAN: Paul Sutton, MD

HISTORY OF PRESENT ILLNESS: The patient is an 18-year-old female who presents to the ED after having a right patellar dislocation. The ambulance was called, and they did easily reduce this. She was playing basketball, rebounded, and landed on her left knee wrong. Denies any ankle or hip pain. In fact, right now she hardly has any knee pain. No previous history of this. General exam showed an 18-year-old female in no acute distress. She had an ice bag on her left knee. No obvious swelling. Patella was nontender to palpation. Full flexion and extension of the knee. No medial or lateral joint line tenderness at the knee. Collateral and cruciate ligaments intact with good end points. X-rays were unremarkable.

ASSESSMENT: Left patellar dislocation, reduced.

PLAN: I discussed my findings and diagnosis with the patient. I told her to buy a Neoprene patellar knee sleeve. Talked with her about strengthening her quads to prevent further injury. I told her she should take it easy the next week and then slowly increase her activity as tolerated.

CPT Code(s): ______________________________

ICD-10-CM Code(s): ______________________________

ICD-9-CM Code(s): ______________________________

Abstracting Questions

1. Does the reduction of the dislocation get reported in addition to the emergency department E/M code?

   ____

2. How many external cause/E codes are reported for this encounter? ______________________________

Case 5-9: Leg Laceration

Assign external cause codes/E codes to indicate how the injury occurred and the place of occurrence. Dr. Sutton is an employee of the hospital.

LOCATION: Outpatient, Hospital

PATIENT: Stone Wilson

PRIMARY CARE PHYSICIAN: Ronald Green, MD

ED PHYSICIAN: Paul Sutton, MD

SUBJECTIVE: This is a 35-year-old male who has no ongoing medical problems, takes no medication. No known allergies. He is up to date for tetanus immunization, having received one last year in December when he cut his hand while trimming the holiday tree. He presents today with a left leg laceration that is 48 hours old.

OBJECTIVE: He has a laceration on his left leg that is healing second intention at this time. There is no evidence of secondary infection presently. This wound was cleaned with saline and Betadine and dressed with Steri-Strips, Bacitracin nonadherent dressing, and a Kling wrap.

ASSESSMENT: Greater than 48-hour right leg laceration, treated as above.

PLAN: Prophylactic Keflex, 500 t.i.d. Follow up for wound check and dressing change in the early part of the next week.

CPT Code(s): ______________________________

ICD-10-CM Code(s): ______________________________

ICD-9-CM Code(s): ______________________________

Abstracting Questions

1. Does the delay in seeking treatment affect the diagnosis code? ______________________
2. Would an external cause code/E code(s) still be reported if the mechanism of injury is not documented?

   ____

Case 5-10: Abdominal Pain and Diarrhea

Dr. Sutton is an employee of the hospital.

LOCATION: Outpatient, Hospital

PATIENT: Maggie Sullivan

PRIMARY CARE PHYSICIAN: Ronald Green, MD

ED PHYSICIAN: Paul Sutton, MD

SUBJECTIVE: The patient is a 32-year-old who presents to the ED with complaints of abdominal pain and diarrhea. She states that she has a history of irritable bowel syndrome. She said she was diagnosed 10 years ago with Crohn's disease. She saw a gastroenterologist in town here 2 years ago, and physician told her that she did not have Crohn's disease. She states she has been having difficulty controlling her stools and has frequent diarrhea. When she feels the urge to go she has to go within a minute or two or she will soil herself. She states she has soiled her underwear several times the last few days. She states she is stressed out right now with her six children and is feeling weak, depressed, and anxious. Her husband is a long-distance truck driver and is seldom home. When he is, they do not get along well, and she is very frustrated about their relationship. He had just returned from a long trip 2 weeks ago, and her symptoms became much worse since that time. No dysuria or frequency. No vomiting. Appetite has been pretty good.

PAST MEDICAL HISTORY: As noted above.

OBJECTIVE: Showed a 32-year-old female who appeared to be in no acute distress. Pulse 88, blood pressure 124/87, 97% sats on room air. HEENT: Unremarkable. Mucous membranes are moist. Neck: Soft and supple. Heart: Regular. Lungs: Clear. Abdomen: Soft. Bowel sounds active throughout. No guarding, no tenderness. Mild tenderness in the left lateral quadrant. No guarding. Rectal exam revealed some brown stool.

LABORATORY: Amylase normal at 27. LFTs normal. Lipase was 3. CBC was normal with a white count as well as hemoglobin and hematocrit. Stool for occult blood was negative. Flat and upright x-rays of the abdomen showed some scattered stool and gas, nonspecific pattern, no free air, no obstructive pattern. Radiologist's report is pending.

ASSESSMENT
1. Diarrhea.
2. Abdominal pain.

PLAN: She was sleeping when I went to review the labs with her. I sent her home with some Bentyl, told her she can take some Imodium, and she will follow up with her physician this week.

CPT Code(s): ____________________

ICD-10-CM Code(s): ____________________

ICD-9-CM Code(s): ____________________

Abstracting Questions

1. What is Crohn's disease? ______________________________

2. What does LFT (reported as normal in the laboratory section) stand for? ______________________________

Case 5-11: Scrotal Bleeding

Dr. Sutton is an employee of the hospital.

LOCATION: Outpatient, Hospital

PATIENT: Dennis Mueller

PRIMARY CARE PHYSICIAN: Ronald Green, MD

ED PHYSICIAN: Paul Sutton, MD

CHIEF COMPLAINT: Bleeding from right scrotum.

HISTORY OF PRESENT ILLNESS: A 49-year-old male who presents with the chief complaint of bleeding from his right scrotum. This started over an hour ago. He is unable to control the bleeding at home and presents because of it. He has had no trauma to the area. He has not bled from this area before. He denies any significant testicular pain.

PAST MEDICAL HISTORY: He does have a history of heart disease and takes aspirin daily. No other blood thinners and no bleeding predisposition.

ALLERGIES: Penicillin.

OBJECTIVE: This is an alert male who appears to be in no acute distress. Blood pressure is 124/87, pulse 77, respirations 20. Examination of his scrotum shows he has a Band-Aid in place. This was removed. There was a very small ooze still present from a bleeding varicosity of his right scrotum. The underlying testicle was nontender, and left testicle was negative to exam.

ASSESSMENT: Bleeding varicosity, right scrotum.

PLAN: We have reapplied a slight pressure dressing on the area. He will be discharged from the ED with advice to leave this in place for the next several days. Should it happen again, he is advised to hold steady pressure for 20 minutes without looking and then apply a Band-Aid. Follow up p.r.n.

CPT Code(s): ______________________________

ICD-10-CM Code(s): ______________________________

ICD-9-CM Code(s): ______________________________

Abstracting Questions

1. What is a varicosity? ______________________________
2. Would you report the scrotal bleeding? ______________________________
3. Why or why would you not report the scrotal bleeding? ______________________________

Case 5-12: Dyspnea and Tachycardia

Dr. Sutton is an employee of the hospital.

LOCATION: Outpatient, Hospital

PATIENT: Pete Barcome

PRIMARY CARE PHYSICIAN: Ronald Green, MD

ED PHYSICIAN: Paul Sutton, MD

SUBJECTIVE: The patient is a 58-year-old male with a history of a recent MI and bypass ×3 months ago. He presents to the ED with complaints of SOB and fast heart rate. He states that resolved by the time paramedics got there. The patient states that he has been in his usual state of health, which has been well. He felt fine going to bed. He woke up about 11 PM and felt a little bit short of breath and sweaty. He immediately took his blood pressure. He states his blood pressure was good (his baseline is 90 systolic). He took his heart rate; it was 80. A short time after, he rechecked it, and it was 83. He waited a few minutes and checked it again, and it was 85. The fourth time he checked it was 87, and because he was nervous that it might keep going up, he called 911. He states that Dr. Elhart has talked to him about putting in an AICD as he has had some fast heart rates before. Actually he states that if his heart rate would have been in the normal range, like the 70s, he would not have even called. Right now he feels pretty good. He did have two sharp chest pains; each one lasted a second or less. It was below the left breast. This was prior to coming in. He has had no other type of chest discomfort. No discomfort in the neck, jaw, or arms. No abdominal pain. He has not had any flu symptoms. He does work out at cardiac rehab on the treadmill three times a week.

PAST MEDICAL HISTORY: Hypertension, arthritis, dyslipidemia, renal calculi, coronary artery disease. He had an inferior wall MI in 1990; occluded a right coronary artery. Decreased injection fraction of 32%. Unstable angina prior to his bypass.

FAMILY HISTORY: ASCVD.

SOCIAL HISTORY: Rancher. Quit smoking 10 years ago. Prior to that he smoked four packs a day. Alcohol, occasional.

REVIEW OF SYSTEMS: No cough, cold, or URI symptoms.

OBJECTIVE: Exam showed a pleasant male in no acute distress. Temperature 37.3. Pulse 83. Blood pressure 102/50. HEENT was grossly unremarkable. Neck: Soft and supple, obese, no adenopathy, no JVD. Heart was regular S1 and S2, no murmur. Lungs were clear throughout. No rales, no wheezing. Abdomen was soft. Bowel sounds active. No guarding. Extremities showed no cyanosis, no edema. The ECG showed a sinus rhythm, rate of 81. No acute ischemic changes noted. Chest x-ray showed external wires from his CABG, cardiomegaly. No old films to compare to. He appears to have a small posterior effusion on the left. Radiology report pending.

ASSESSMENT
1. Dyspnea.
2. Tachycardia.
3. Status post recent coronary artery bypass.

PLAN: As noted above, when the patient arrived here at 12:01 AM he was feeling back to normal. We discharged him here at 1:05 AM, and during the whole time he felt fine. His blood pressure was in his baseline range, and I had him walk around the ED here a little bit, and he was feeling fine.

Discussed the findings and diagnosis with the patient. He felt comfortable in going home. If he has any further problems, he will return to the ED for follow-up clinic depending on symptoms.

CPT Code(s): ______________________________

ICD-10-CM Code(s): ______________________________

ICD-9-CM Code(s): ______________________________

Abstracting Questions

1. Should the patient's status post coronary artery bypass be reported? ______________________________
2. What does AICD stand for? ______________________________

Chapter 6
Medicine

Make sure to check evolve learning system for the latest content updates

Case 6-1: Echocardiogram

Remember to report only the profession portion of the service when the physician is not an employee of the facility in which the service is being provided.

ECHOCARDIOGRAM REPORT

LOCATION: Outpatient, Hospital

PATIENT: Loralee Branigan

ATTENDING/ADMIT PHYSICIAN: James Noonar, MD

RADIOLOGIST: Morton Monson, MD

PERSONAL PHYSICIAN: Ronald Green, MD

INDICATIONS: Valvular heart disease, atrial fibrillation, left ventricular dysfunction.

The M-Mode echo measurements are listed on the accompanying data sheet. They are essentially within normal limits.

The two-dimensional echocardiogram clearly demonstrates some thickening and calcification of the mitral valve leaflets as well as thickening of the aortic valve leaflets. The aortic valve opening is normal, and the mitral valve opening is probably normal as well. Left ventricular contractility is definitely diminished. The ejection fraction is in the range of about 20-25% only.

The Doppler and color Doppler studies do confirm the presence of mild tricuspid insufficiency. The RV systolic pressure is 32 mm Hg, which is consistent with mild pulmonary hypertension.

CONCLUSION: Depression of left ventricular function, as described above, with mild valvular pathology, as described above.

CPT Code(s): ______________________________

ICD-10-CM Code(s): ______________________________

ICD-9-CM Code(s): ______________________________

Abstracting Questions

1. What approach was used for the cardiac echocardiogram? ______________________
2. Is the Doppler study also reported? ______________________
3. Is the Doppler color flow study reported? ______________________
4. What modifier is required on the CPT code? ______________________

Case 6-2: Stress Test

STRESS TEST REPORT

LOCATION: Outpatient, Hospital

PATIENT: Troy Carlos

REQUESTING PHYSICIAN: Frank Gaul, MD

PHYSICIAN: David Barton, MD

INDICATION: Preoperative assessment for amputation. The patient has a history of aortic and mitral valve replacement.

BASELINE DATA: Blood pressure is 100/43. Heart rate 76. Baseline ECG reveals 100% ventricular pacing.

STRESS: The patient was injected with 67.2 mg adenosine over 6 minutes. At 3 minutes the patient was injected with Myoview. The patient had nonspecific complaints. Heart rate did not change from baseline. Blood pressure nadir was 80/36. The patient was reversed with 250 mg aminophylline and was discharged in stable condition and remained paced.

CONCLUSION
1. Borderline vasodilator response by adenosine.
2. Inconclusive adenosine for inducible ischemia by ECG criteria secondary to the presence of 100% ventricular pacing.
3. Myoview is pending.

CPT Code(s): ____________________

ICD-10-CM Code(s): ____________________

ICD-9-CM Code(s): ____________________

Abstracting Questions

1. What services need to be reported for the physician? ____________________
2. What was the reason for the encounter? ____________________
3. Are Z/V codes the only diagnoses reported for this case? ____________________

Case 6-3: Cardiac Catheterization

CARDIAC CATHETERIZATION REPORT

LOCATION: Inpatient, Hospital

PATIENT: Wade Land

REFERRING PHYSICIAN: James Noonar, MD

CARDIOLOGIST: Marvin Elhart, MD

INDICATION: Unstable angina.

PROCEDURE: Right iliofemoral angiography, left heart catheterization, selective coronary angiography, and left ventriculography.

COMPLICATIONS: None.

RESULTS: Hemodynamics: The left ventricular pressure before the LV gram was 133/7 with an LVEDP of 11. After the LV gram it was 130/8 with an LVEDP of 12. The aortic pressure on pullback was 130/59.

Left Ventriculography: Showed that the left ventricle is normal in size. It was hard to assess segmental wall motion because of the frequency of PVCs; however, the overall left ventricular systolic function was normal. There might be some distal anterior wall hypokinesis.

Selective Coronary Angiography

1. Right coronary artery: This was a medium-size dominant artery that has mild diffuse atherosclerotic changes. After the PDA there was about 30% narrowing.
2. Left main coronary artery: This has 80-90% eccentric narrowing in the midportion.
3. Left circumflex artery: This was a medium-size artery that has mild atherosclerotic changes proximally. It gave rise to a medium-size bifurcating first obtuse marginal that has 99% proximal narrowing. The inferior of the two branches, which was a smaller size artery, has 90% proximal narrowing.
4. Left anterior descending coronary artery: This was a medium-size artery that has mild diffuse atherosclerotic changes. The first diagonal was a small artery that had 90% proximal narrowing. The second diagonal was a larger artery that has about 60% narrowing in the midportion. Immediately after that diagonal, the left anterior descending artery has about 50% narrowing. There was moderate diffuse disease after that. Please note that the visualization of the diagonals and the left anterior descending artery was rather limited as we tried not to inject in a strong way into the left main.

CONCLUSION

1. Normal overall left ventricular systolic function.
2. Severe left main disease.
3. Severe left circumflex and first diagonal disease.

RECOMMENDATIONS

1. Maximum medical treatment.
2. Intra-aortic balloon pump.
3. Consult CT surgery to evaluate the patient for bypass surgery.

CPT Code(s): ____________________

ICD-10-CM Code(s): ____________________

ICD-9-CM Code(s): ____________________

Abstracting Questions

1. What are the three categories bundled into the code reported for cardiac catheterization? ____________
2. What was the approach for this procedure? ____________
3. Was a modifier required on the catheterization code and if a modifier was required, which one would it be? ____________
4. For what two procedures were injections provided? ____________

Case 6-4: Cardiac Catheterization

CARDIAC CATHETERIZATION REPORT

LOCATION: Inpatient, Hospital

PATIENT: Jo Littledove

REFERRING PHYSICIAN: James Noonar, MD

CARDIOLOGIST: Marvin Elhart, MD

INDICATIONS: Abnormal Cardiolite stress test and shortness of breath.

PROCEDURE: Right and left selective coronary angiogram, LV gram left heart, right femoral artery #6 French sheath, right femoral artery angiogram.

HEMODYNAMICS: Aortic pressure 138/57, LV 148/4. No aortic gradient on pullback.

RESULTS: Ventriculography: The LV displayed normal size with excellent contractility and no segmental wall motion abnormality. The ejection fraction is estimated at 60-80%.

Coronary Angiography

1. Right coronary artery: This is a dominant vessel. It has a shepherd's crook takeoff. Through its course the right coronary artery has no significant stenosis. Distally, it trifurcated to give rise to posterior descending artery, posterolateral branch, and a marginal branch. Through its course the right coronary artery has intimal disease from 10-20%.
2. Left main: Normal.
3. Circumflex artery: The circumflex artery is a codominant system. The circumflex in its midportion branched to give first marginal that is moderate in size, tortuous, but no significant obstructive disease, and a very large second marginal that has in its midportion 40% stenosis. Distally, it branched to give smaller marginals.
4. Left anterior descending artery: After the takeoff of the left main, has steep angulations of close to 90 degrees. Thereafter it takes off and through its course has significant tortuosity. The proximal part of the left anterior descending appears slightly hazy, probably from the angulations; the artery itself has 30% stenosis. At the level of the stenosis there are two diagonals taking off, the first of which is before the stenosis and is small, and the second one is moderate in size and has at its origin an ostial stenosis that appeared to be 60%. The left anterior descending artery is tortuous and in its midportion gave rise to another diagonal that appeared to be free of any significant disease.

IMPRESSION/CONCLUSION: Normal left ventricular systolic functions with disease involving predominantly the left anterior descending artery that appeared to be in its proximal third of 40-50% at the level of the second diagonal. Angiographically, it did not appear severely obstructed, with some mild disease involving the right coronary artery at the circumflex. At this point, my recommendation is to aggressively manage her medically, and if we are unable to control her symptoms with medications, then later on we might consider percutaneous revascularization of the left anterior descending artery. Considering her size, the location of the lesion, and the takeoff of the left anterior descending artery, this procedure is not without risk.

CPT Code(s): ______________________________

ICD-10-CM Code(s): ______________________________

ICD-9-CM Code(s): ______________________________

Abstracting Questions

1. What does the LV referred to in the report stand for? ______________________________
2. What is the definition of "circumflex"? ______________________________
3. The report states in point 4 that the left anterior descending artery has significant tortuosity. What does this mean? ______________________________

Case 6-5: Right Heart Catheterization

REPORT OF OPERATION

LOCATION: Inpatient, Hospital

PATIENT: Beth Ritter

ATTENDING/ADMIT PHYSICIAN: Frank Gaul, MD

SURGEON: James Noonar, MD

PREOPERATIVE DIAGNOSIS: Diabetes insipidus. Difficulty with IV access plus difficulty with fluid balance.

POSTOPERATIVE DIAGNOSIS: Diabetes insipidus. Difficulty with IV access plus difficulty with fluid balance.

PROCEDURE PERFORMED: Right heart catheterization with Swan-Ganz catheter.

PROCEDURE: After Betadine scrub to the right subclavian vein area and the internal jugular Swan was removed, the area was then anesthetized with 8 cc of 1% lidocaine. Once this was accomplished with a one-pass maneuver, the subclavian vein was cannulated. Once that was in place, the guidewire was inserted through the needle. The needle was removed, and then the tissue dilator and sheath were pushed into position over the guidewire. Once this was in position, the wire and the tissue dilator were removed and the Swan-Ganz catheter advanced. The CVP pressure and RA pressure were 7, RV pressure was 36/5, mean of 18, PA pressure was 35/18, mean of 23, and wedge pressure was 10. We will get a cardiac index output later, and we will check a chest x-ray to make sure we have good placement.

There was scant bleeding and no observable complications.

CPT Code(s): ______________________________

ICD-10-CM Code(s): ______________________________

ICD-9-CM Code(s): ______________________________

Abstracting Questions

1. Does the Swan-Ganz for monitoring affect the CPT code assignment? ______________________________
2. Was the removal of the Swan from the internal jugular reported? ______________________________

Case 6-6: Bilateral Laser–Doppler

RADIOLOGY REPORT

LOCATION: Outpatient, Hospital

PATIENT: Gordon Monday

ORDERING PHYSICIAN: Laddie N. Noss, MD

ATTENDING/ADMIT PHYSICIAN: Laddie N. Noss, MD

RADIOLOGIST: Morton Monson, MD

PERSONAL PHYSICIAN: Ronald Green, MD

EXAMINATION: Bilateral laser-Doppler test.

CLINICAL SYMPTOMS: Ischemic left toe due to PVD.

BILATERAL LASER-DOPPLER TEST: The patient is an 84-year-old man with diabetes and renal disease. He had an arterial Doppler 6 months previously that showed bilateral disease and calcified vessels. The right side showed a digital pressure of 70. The left side was more abnormal with a digital pressure of only 12. Again, vessels were calcified.

On the left side, the toe pressure is 35, which is right at the borderline of healing. Transmetatarsal is at the same level. Above the ankle, paradoxically, the pressure is even a little lower at 30, which is right at our threshold. On the right side at the toe, the level is 70, which indicates a good likelihood of healing. Transmetatarsal the level is 60 and above the ankle is 50, all of which should be adequate for healing.

The laser-Doppler studies basically back up the digit pressures. The right side looks abnormal, but adequate for healing. The left side is marginal. Laser-Doppler levels look a little better than the digit pressures regarding this area.

CPT Code(s): ______________________________

ICD-10-CM Code(s): ______________________________

ICD-9-CM Code(s): ______________________________

Abstracting Questions

1. Does the laser description affect the CPT code selection for the Doppler scan? ______________
2. Was CPT code selection affected by arterial or venous study? ______________
3. Does bilateral versus unilateral affect CPT assignment? ______________

Case 6-7: Saphenous Vein Mapping

RADIOLOGY REPORT

LOCATION: Outpatient, Hospital

PATIENT: Mirta Hubert

ORDERING PHYSICIAN: James Noonar, MD

ATTENDING/ADMIT PHYSICIAN: James Noonar, MD

RADIOLOGIST: Morton Monson, MD

PERSONAL PHYSICIAN: Alma Naraquist, MD

EXAMINATION: Saphenous vein mapping.

CLINICAL SYMPTOMS: Pre-coronary artery bypass graft; atherosclerotic heart disease of native coronary arteries, chest pain.

FINDINGS: The left greater saphenous vein was mapped from midthigh through the proximal calf. Measurements above the knee were 1.0 × 0.92 cm, at the knee 0.73 × 0.73 cm, and below the knee 0.54 × 0.54 cm. The multiple branches encountered were not evaluated.

CPT Code(s): ______________________________

ICD-10-CM Code(s): ______________________________

ICD-9-CM Code(s): ______________________________

Abstracting Questions

1. What type of scan was used for mapping of vessels? ______________________________

Case 6-8: Venous Ultrasound

RADIOLOGY REPORT

LOCATION: Inpatient, Hospital

PATIENT: Dave James

ORDERING PHYSICIAN: Frank Gaul, MD

ATTENDING/ADMIT PHYSICIAN: Frank Gaul, MD

RADIOLOGIST: Morton Monson, MD

PERSONAL PHYSICIAN: Frank Gaul, MD

EXAMINATION: Bilateral lower extremity venous ultrasound.

CLINICAL SYMPTOMS: Leg pain and swelling. Rule out deep venous thrombosis.

FINDINGS: This examination was somewhat limited as a result of the patient being recently out of surgery and unable to be moved at all. As visualized, both the right and the left common femoral, superficial femoral, popliteal, and posterior tibial veins are fully compressible and demonstrate the presence of normal spontaneous, phasic, and augmented flow.

IMPRESSION: No evidence for deep venous thrombosis is seen within either of the lower extremities. Please see above comments.

CPT Code(s): ______________________________

ICD-10-CM Code(s): ______________________________

ICD-9-CM Code(s): ______________________________

Abstracting Questions

1. What is a deep venous thrombosis? ______________________________

Case 6-9: Extremities Ultrasound

RADIOLOGY REPORT

LOCATION: Outpatient, Hospital

PATIENT: Eric Tayes

ORDERING PHYSICIAN: Frank Gaul, MD

ATTENDING/ADMIT PHYSICIAN: Frank Gaul, MD

RADIOLOGIST: Morton Monson, MD

EXAMINATION: Ultrasound of both lower extremities; abdomen ultrasound.

CLINICAL SYMPTOMS: Lower extremity swelling, difficulty breathing.

FINDINGS: Ultrasound examination of the deep venous system of both lower extremities is negative. No evidence of deep venous thrombosis in either lower extremity. The posterior tibial, greater saphenous, and popliteal through the femoral veins are patent and negative for thrombus bilaterally. Normal phasicity.

Abdomen Ultrasound: Diffusely coarsened echotexture of the liver with some nodularity consistent with fatty infiltration. Cirrhotic configuration of the liver. Small calcified granuloma in the spleen. The spleen is otherwise negative. There is ascites in all four quadrants. No bile duct dilatation. No gallbladder wall thickening or cholelithiasis. Small amount of fluid adjacent to the gallbladder is likely related to the ascites. The pancreas is obscured by bowel gas. The abdominal aorta is of normal caliber. The right kidney measures approximately 9 cm in length and shows no evidence of hydronephrosis, calculi, or mass. The left kidney measures approximately 9.9 cm in length and shows no evidence of hydronephrosis, calculi, or mass.

CPT Code(s): ______________________________

ICD-10-CM Code(s): ______________________________

ICD-9-CM Code(s): ______________________________

Abstracting Questions

1. How was the scan for the abdomen different than the scan for the extremities? ______________
2. How would the "cirrhotic configuration of the liver" diagnosis be reported? ______________

Case 6-10: Renal Dialysis Progress Note

RENAL DIALYSIS PROGRESS NOTE

LOCATION: Outpatient, Clinic

PATIENT: Jyl Couts

PHYSICIAN: Ira Avila, MD

The 45-year-old patient presents today for regular monthly visit. She has been slightly tired. She denies any shortness of breath or chest pain. No constipation. The patient complains of some weakness in her legs when she walks to the grocery store.

PHYSICAL EXAMINATION: Her blood pressure at home has been in the 130s/80s. On exam today, her weight is 152.5 pounds. Regular heart rate at 79 per minute. The lungs are clear bilaterally without crackles. No edema in the extremities. Catheter condition is good, and the exit site is clean and dry. No evidence of infection.

IMPRESSION/PLAN

1. The patient is on CAPD, two bag sizes of 1.5% and 2.5%; doing well with that.
2. She is on 4000 units of EPO once a week due to anemia due to end-stage renal disease with hemoglobin of 12. We will continue that at this time.
3. The patient has possibility of claudication. She has history of an aneurysm, which was measured at 6.1 cm on a CT scan done in the transverse section. We will obtain an ultrasound to follow up on her abdominal aortic aneurysm and do ABIs on the lower extremities.
4. The patient requested a handicap permit, and I will hold that for now until we do her studies.

The patient seems to agree with the plan.

CPT Code(s): ________________________________

ICD-10-CM Code(s): ________________________________

ICD-9-CM Code(s): ________________________________

Abstracting Questions

1. Does the type of dialysis the patient receives affect code selection? ____________________
2. What is end-stage renal disease? ________________________________

Chapter 7
Gastroenterology

Case 7-1: Orogastric Tube Placement

OPERATIVE REPORT

The intraoperative KUB was provided by the radiologist, and you are only reporting the services of Dr. Friendly.

LOCATION: Outpatient, Hospital

PATIENT: Otto Garth

ATTENDING/ADMIT PHYSICIAN: Alma Naraquist, MD

SURGEON: Larry P. Friendly, MD

INDICATION: Feeding, patient with gastroparesis.

PROCEDURE: The patient was placed in the sitting position and then tilted to the right with a wedge. CORFLO was placed at the level of 19 cm without any complications. KUB was then done demonstrating the tip of the CORFLO in the third portion of the duodenum. After confirmation of postpyloric position of the CORFLO, the patient was started on UltraCal at 10 cc/hour.

CPT Code(s): ______________________________

ICD-10-CM Code(s): ______________________________

ICD-9-CM Code(s): ______________________________

Abstracting Questions

1. What does KUB stand for? ______________________________
2. What type of tube is a CORFLO? ______________________________

Case 7-2: Splenectomy and Colectomy

OPERATIVE REPORT

LOCATION: Inpatient, Hospital

PATIENT: Sara Milton

ATTENDING/ADMIT PHYSICIAN: Alma Naraquist, MD

SURGEON: Larry P. Friendly, MD

PREOPERATIVE DIAGNOSIS: Abdominal sepsis.

POSTOPERATIVE DIAGNOSIS: Myeloproliferative disorder; sigmoid perforation, pleural effusion, abdominal sepsis.

PROCEDURES PERFORMED
1. Exploratory laparotomy with splenectomy.
2. Sigmoid colectomy with the Hartmann procedure and mobilization of the splenic flexure.
3. Tru-Cut biopsy of liver times two.
4. Placement of right #28 French chest tube.

ANESTHESIA: General.

INDICATIONS: The patient is a 69-year-old female admitted with abdominal pain this past Friday. CT scan showed an infarction of a very large spleen. Over the weekend, she developed increasing pain, then required fluid resuscitation and was found to have question of free air on upright abdominal x-ray. Her abdominal examination was consistent with intraperitoneal catastrophe, and we discussed operative intervention, including splenectomy, possible bowel resection, possible colostomy, and placement of a right-sided chest tube for a very large right pleural effusion, with the patient and her husband. They understood this and wished to proceed.

PROCEDURE: The patient was brought down to the operating room and placed under general anesthesia after an A-line and right CVP line were placed by anesthesia. A midline incision was made with a #10 blade, and dissection was carried down through subcutaneous tissues using electrocautery. The subcutaneous tissue was very edematous. We divided the midline fascia and then opened the peritoneum sharply, allowing entry into the peritoneal cavity. There was hemorrhagic fluid within the peritoneal cavity. We could see a very large spleen. We took down the phrenic attachments as well as the splenic flexure, the peritoneal attachments between right angle clamps, and then identified the splenic vein and splenic artery, and doubly tied these proximally and singly tied them distally before dividing them. We then removed the spleen and sent it to pathology for frozen section, where it was consistent with some type of myeloproliferative disorder going on. We ran the bowel, and the sigmoid colon was attached to the mesentery of the proximal jejunum. There was a hematoma here that had ruptured, and in dissecting the hematoma free we could see a small perforation in the sigmoid colon. We debrided the mesentery, debrided the mesenteric abscess, and then divided the sigmoid mesentery between right angle clamps and tied the vascular pedicles with 2–0 silk free ties. We fired a TLC-75 stapler distally across the distal sigmoid colon and then mobilized the splenic flexure and fired it proximally across the descending colon. We sent the sigmoid out for permanent section. After we had freely mobilized the splenic flexure and debrided the abscess cavity, we irrigated with saline until returns were clear. We did two Tru-Cut needle biopsies of the left lobe of the liver and controlled bleeding with electrocautery. The remainder of the bowel appeared normal. We then made a stomal opening in the left lower quadrant by grasping the skin with a Kocher clamp, excising it in an elliptical fashion, dividing the anterior and posterior sheath in cruciate fashion, and delivering the descending colon through the stomal opening. We then closed the midline fascia with a combination of interrupted 0 Vicryl and running 0 PDS. The skin was closed loosely with a few skin clips. We then secured the colon with 3–0 Vicryl sutures. The colon appeared viable. Also the small bowel, which had appeared patchy at first, was quite viable when we had completed the procedure. We then prepped the right chest and we made an incision with a #11 blade. We carried our dissection up over the top of approximately the fourth or the fifth ribs, entered the pleural space with a Kelly clamp, dilated the tract with a Kelly clamp, and then placed a #28 French chest tube. We returned about 900 cc of bloody fluid from the chest. We secured this in place, hooked it up to -20 cm of water suction, and then dressed it. The patient was then left intubated and taken to the surgical critical care unit in critical but stable condition.

CPT Code(s): ____________________

ICD-10-CM Code(s): ____________________

ICD-9-CM Code(s): ____________________

Abstracting Questions

1. Is the exploratory laparotomy reported separately? ____________________
2. Does the Hartmann procedure affect the selection of the colectomy code? ____________________
3. Were the procedures performed open or closed? ____________________
4. Would "mobilization of splenic flexure" be reported separately? ____________________
5. Does the "separate procedure" designation affect the splenectomy CPT code selection? ____________________
6. What type of biopsy is a Tru-Cut liver biopsy? ____________________
7. What procedure was reported with a CPT code that required a modifier or modifiers to be appended to the code? ____________________
8. Was the anesthesia provided during the procedure general anesthesia? ____________________

Case 7-3: Gastrojejunostomy Placement

Because this is an interventional radiologist performing the procedure, you report both the procedure and the radiology services.

RADIOLOGY REPORT

LOCATION: Outpatient, Hospital

PATIENT: Betty Frye

ORDERING PHYSICIAN: Ronald Green, MD

ATTENDING/ADMIT PHYSICIAN: Ronald Green, MD

INTERVENTIONAL RADIOLOGIST: Monica Hamilton, MD

EXAMINATION: Gastrojejunostomy placement.

CLINICAL SYMPTOMS: Malnutrition needing nutritional support.

INDICATION: The patient is a 69-year-old female requiring tube feeding. Placement of a #14 French Shetty gastrojejunostomy catheter was requested by Dr. Green for nutritional support.

Prior to the start of the study, the procedure was explained to the patient, including the risks, complications, and alternatives. The patient understood and consented to the procedure.

PERCUTANEOUS GASTROJEJUNOSTOMY PLACEMENT: The patient was prepped and draped in the usual sterile fashion. Using ultrasound guidance, we localized the edge of the liver. Through a previously placed nasogastric tube, the stomach was distended with air.

Using fluoroscopic guidance following administration of local anesthesia (1% lidocaine), we performed gastropexy utilizing four Medi-Tech T-tacks at the mid to distal aspect of the stomach.

Using multiple wires and catheters, an extra-stiff guidewire was ultimately placed with the tip in the proximal jejunum. Following multiple dilatations, a #14 French Shetty gastrojejunostomy catheter was placed with the tip in the proximal jejunum. A small amount of contrast was administered, which revealed adequate placement. There is no evidence of extravasation or other significant abnormalities.

The patient tolerated the procedure well. There was no evidence of bleeding at the termination of the study.

IMPRESSION: Placement of a #14 French Shetty gastrojejunostomy catheter with the tip in the proximal jejunum, as described above.

CPT Code(s): ______________________________

ICD-10-CM Code(s): ______________________________

ICD-9-CM Code(s): ______________________________

Abstracting Questions

1. What was the approach for insertion of the gastrostomy tube? ____________________
2. Was the ultrasonic guidance separately reported? ____________________
3. Was the radiology service to check placement separately reported? ____________________

Case 7-4: Cystotomy

OPERATIVE REPORT

Dr. Martinez operated on this patient yesterday. The patient presents to the emergency department with an acute abdomen. You are to report only Dr. Martinez's services.

LOCATION: Inpatient, Hospital

PATIENT: Patti Bryan

ATTENDING PHYSICIAN: Gary Sanchez, MD

SURGEONS: Paula Smithson, MD, and Andy Martinez, MD

PREOPERATIVE DIAGNOSES
1. Acute abdomen.
2. Hematuria with suspected bladder injury.

POSTOPERATIVE DIAGNOSES
1. Iatrogenic cystotomy with urine extravasation into the peritoneal cavity.
2. Peritonitis.
3. Extensive intestinal adhesions.

PROCEDURES PERFORMED
1. Exploratory laparotomy.
2. Closure of cystotomy.
3. Extensive intestinal adhesiolysis.

SURGICAL INDICATIONS: This patient is a 32-year-old female who had undergone a Hasson laparoscopy that I performed yesterday. She presented to the emergency department last night with abdominal pain and findings of an acute abdomen. She also had a leukopenia. She was not running a fever. She was noted on insertion of the catheter into the bladder to have some grossly bloody urine.

OPERATIVE FINDINGS: There was less than 1-cm laceration in the dome of the bladder that was extravasating through the bladder. There was a large amount of urine in the peritoneal cavity and some slightly foul-smelling purulent fluid as well. This looked relatively murky and was just not plain urine. There were multiple intestinal adhesions, mostly involving the small bowel. No perforation of the bowel could be detected. The appendix was normal.

OPERATIVE DESCRIPTION: After induction of general anesthesia with patient in the supine position, the abdomen was prepped and draped. The abdomen was opened through a midline hypogastric incision excising her old scar on the way in. The above findings were noted initially, and Dr. Smithson was able to isolate the small bladder dome laceration. This was smaller than one would expect if a 5-mm laparoscopic trocar had gone through the bladder. I believe that the edge of the bladder probably was nicked. Dr. Smithson will dictate her note concerning the cystotomy repair. We then ran the bowel in its entirety from the ligament of Treitz on down to the ileocecal junction. There were multiple interloop adhesions, which were lysed by Dr. Smithson. She will dictate her note separately. Some omental adhesions were also lysed. After copious irrigation of the abdominal cavity, we then irrigated with heparinized lactated Ringer's and left some of the Ringer's in the abdomen. The peritoneum was closed with a running 2–0 Vicryl. The fascia was closed with interrupted figure-of-eight 0 Vicryl, and the skin closed with staples. Blood loss estimation was 100 cc. The patient received 3000 cc of lactated Ringer's during the case.

Specimens to pathology were cultures of the peritoneal fluid. A Foley catheter was changed at the end of the case. The patient was returned to the recovery room in stable condition.

CPT Code(s): ______________________________

ICD-10-CM Code(s): ______________________________

ICD-9-CM Code(s): ______________________________

Abstracting Questions

1. What procedures were performed during this operative session? ______________________________
2. Which of the procedures did Dr. Martinez perform? ______________________________
3. Were any modifiers required for the two surgeons involved in the same session and if so, which modifier?

   ____

Case 7-5: Small-Bowel Anastomosis

OPERATIVE REPORT

LOCATION: Inpatient, Hospital

PATIENT: Dona Kelly

ATTENDING PHYSICIAN: Ronald Green, MD

SURGEON: Daniel G. Olanka, MD

PREOPERATIVE DIAGNOSIS: Multiple intestinal fistulas.

POSTOPERATIVE DIAGNOSIS: Multiple intestinal fistulas.

PROCEDURE PERFORMED: Excision of abdominal wall and small bowel with primary anastomosis of small bowel.

PRELIMINARY NOTE: This patient is well known to us. She has had multiple abdominal procedures to try to repair a very large abdominal wall hernia. She is outside the postoperative period of the hernia repair. She basically has no abdominal cavity left, and all her intestine resides outside the abdomen. There is such a drag on her abdominal wall that she has developed fistulas at the base of where the bowel rests against the mesh, and these have become unmanageable in the home setting. On this basis, we take this very high-risk patient to the operating room, with appropriate counseling for the family about the dire consequences.

OPERATIVE NOTE: With the patient under general anesthesia, the abdomen was prepped and draped in a sterile manner. A long incision was made above the area of the fistulas, and we began to work our way down onto the mesh. Unfortunately, we entered the bowel at multiple points and had multiple enterotomies into the small bowel *(small intestine)* and colon *(large intestine)*. Finally we got everything freed up and were able to resect some of the abdominal wall that had adherent small bowel to it *(this indicates that part of the small intestine was removed)*. We were able to repair all of the enterostomies and a right colotomy using two layers of suture, an inner layer of Vicryl, and an outer layer of silk. We then copiously irrigated the abdominal field and used some large retention-type sutures to bring the wound together for partial closure. It is our hopes that the bowel that remains is viable *(this indicates that part of the bowel was removed)*. This procedure took substantially greater time than typically would be required. *(This statement indicates -22 may be assigned.)* We measured it at approximately 200 cm of length of her small bowel, and we are hopeful that this will be enough for her to nourish adequately.

CPT Code(s): ______________________________

ICD-10-CM Code(s): ______________________________

ICD-9-CM Code(s): ______________________________

Abstracting Questions

1. Was a portion of the large or small intestine removed?______________________________
2. What statement indicates that modifier -22 would be appended to the CPT code?______________________________

Case 7-6: Pyloroplasty

OPERATIVE REPORT

Report only Dr. White's surgical services. Note in this case that the surgeon began the procedure as a percutaneous liver biopsy, but because the patient could not hold his breath long enough for the biopsy to be obtained, Dr. White decided to discontinue the percutaneous biopsy and take the patient directly to the operating room for an open procedure. Two surgeons (co-surgeons) are performing this case. Dr. Sanchez, in his operative report, states that the patient was turned to a lateral position, prepped, and draped and the chest was opened to expose the esophagus. The distal esophagus was mobilized under direct vision and divided above the diseased segment. The distal esophagus and the attached proximal stomach were removed. The remaining stomach was pulled into the chest and connected to the stump of the proximal esophagus. Drains were placed and a chest tube inserted and the incision was closed.

LOCATION: Inpatient, Hospital

PATIENT: Ted Boyd

ATTENDING PHYSICIAN: Larry Friendly, MD

PRIMARY CARE PHYSICIAN: Ronald Green, MD

SURGEONS: Loren White, MD, and Gary Sanchez, MD

PREOPERATIVE DIAGNOSIS: Barrett's esophagus with severe dysplasia, possible carcinoma.

POSTOPERATIVE DIAGNOSIS: Barrett's esophagus with severe dysplasia, possible carcinoma, hemangioma liver.

PROCEDURES PERFORMED
1. Exploratory laparotomy.
2. Biopsy of liver lesion.
3. Immobilization of stomach with pyloroplasty.
4. Placement of feeding tube.

PRELIMINARY NOTE: This patient is a 63-year-old man who has been referred by Dr. Green for a bleeding esophageal lesion. This was seen and scoped, and the patient was markedly anemic. Biopsies showed it to be severe dysplasia with possible cancer present. He has had a rather extensive workup including complete cardiac workup. CT of the abdomen showed some lesions within the liver, which we tried to have biopsied percutaneously, but the patient could not hold his breath well enough and the lesions were too close to the diaphragm, so we do not have a tissue diagnosis on these. After all this workup we are taking the patient to the operating room for exploration. Assuming that he does not have disease metastatic to the liver, we will proceed with an esophagogastrectomy in the Ivor-Lewis technique. The abdominal portion of the procedure, which I am dictating, will be done by myself, and then Dr. Sanchez will do the chest portion of the procedure.

OPERATIVE NOTE: With the patient under general anesthesia, the abdomen was prepped and draped in a sterile manner. Midline incision was made from the xiphoid to below the pubis. Sharp dissection was carried down into the peritoneal cavity, and hemostasis was maintained with electrocautery. We began by exploring the abdominal cavity. The liver was carefully palpated. The area that had been identified on CT was at the very apex of the right lobe of the liver, we could feel this area; it did not have a thickened feel to it but was more consistent with an area of hemangioma. There was a small secondary lesion on the undersurface of the right lobe. A **wedge biopsy** of this was taken and it did return a diagnosis of hemangioma. The rest of the liver appeared normal, and I thought that we did not need to proceed with anything further. We thus began with mobilization of the stomach, taking down the greater curvature vessels, preserving the gastroepiploica. We carried our dissection all the way up into the hiatal hernia, preserving the blood supply to the spleen and not injuring it. We were then able to detach the left gastric artery such that the stomach was tethered on its other vasculature but appeared completely viable. All these vessels were taken down with clamps and ligatures of 2–0 silk. We then circumferentially went around the esophagus and carried our dissection all the way back toward the pylorus. We then had the entire stomach freed up from pylorus all the way up to the diaphragm. *(The esophagus has been mobilized where it passes through the diaphragm and the stomach has been totally freed up so that when the chest is opened Dr. Sanchez will perform the remaining part of the surgery.)* The stomach appeared viable with reasonable circulation. A Heineke-Mikulicz **pyloroplasty** was then performed opening the pylorus in one direction and closing it in another using interrupted 3–0 silk sutures to complete the pyloroplasty. With this accomplished, we then picked up the **jejunum** approximated 40 or 50 cm beyond the ligament of Treitz and placed a red rubber **feeding tube** using a Witzel technique; this was a number 18-2. This was attached to the skin and brought out through a separate stab incision. The abdominal cavity was then checked for hemostasis and everything appeared to be intact. We then closed the incision using running 0–loop nylon. We closed the skin with staples. A sterile dressing was applied. With all this completed, the patient remained in the operating room and will be positioned by Dr. Sanchez for the thoracic portion of the procedure.

Pathology Report Later Indicated: Hemangioma.

CPT Code(s): ____________________

ICD-10-CM Code(s): ____________________

ICD-9-CM Code(s): ____________________

Abstracting Questions

1. Can the discontinued percutaneous liver biopsy be reported? ____________________
2. If reporting the percutaneous liver biopsy, what modifier(s) is/are required? ____________________
3. Was the wedge biopsy reported? ____________________
4. Dr. White performed an immobilization and what other procedure? ____________________
5. Was the Barrett's and hemangioma reported separately? ____________________

Chapter 8
Nephrology

Make sure to check evolve learning system for the latest content updates

Case 8-1: Progress Note, Dialysis

PROGRESS NOTE

LOCATION: Inpatient, Hospital

PATIENT: Monica Garcia

ATTENDING PHYSICIAN: George Orbitz, MD

The patient is seen and examined. The chart is reviewed. The patient appears to be hemodynamically stable and not in any form of respiratory distress or compromise. Her complaint mainly centers on her bilateral lower extremity edema, for which I have advised elevation of the lower extremities. It must be recalled that we have withheld all diuretics and ACE inhibitors in this particular patient as she has been intravenously volume depleted for the past several days.

PHYSICAL EXAMINATION: Vital signs are stable. Blood pressure is 110/50s. Heart rate is 80s. Respirations are 20s. Saturating well above 90% on room air. She is afebrile. She has had urine output between 1 and 2 liters in the last 24 hours. Normocephalic and atraumatic with pink palpebral conjunctivae and anicteric sclerae. No nasal or aural discharge. Moist tongue and buccal mucosa. No pharyngeal hyperemia, congestion, or exudates. Neck is supple. No lymphadenopathy. Symmetric chest expansion. No retractions. No rhonchi. No crackles or wheezes. S1 and S2 are distinct. No S3 or S4. Regular rate and rhythm. Abdomen: Positive bowel sounds; soft and nontender. Both upper and lower extremities reveal arthritic changes. Positive edema on both lower extremities. Pulses are fair.

Latest laboratory tests on this patient are as follows: Sodium 138, potassium 4.3, chloride 107, CO_2 18.7, BUN and creatinine are 52/2.3 (67/3.8 on March 16; 76/5.1 on March 15; 76/5.4 on March 14—initial consultation), glucose 96, calcium 8.5, magnesium 1.4, phosphorus 4.0, albumin 2.7. Hemogram shows hemoglobin and hematocrit of 10/29.9, WBC 11.01, normochromic/normocytic indices, and platelets 170.

ASSESSMENT/PLAN

1. Acute renal failure, significantly improved. Most likely secondary to intravascular volume depletion brought about by overzealous use of diuretics, decreased p.o. intake, nausea, and vomiting. Once again, this condition has significantly improved as her creatinine is now down, too. Likewise, BUN is also significantly decreased. At this time, I would recommend to continue IV fluid hydration for another day while monitoring inputs and outputs and daily weights closely. Because the acute problem of azotemia has significantly resolved and

the patient is on an improving trend, at this time I am going to sign off the case. Patient would benefit from following up with outpatient nephrology/Dr. Orbitz within the next 1 to 2 weeks.

2. Chronic renal failure (latest creatinine clearance is 21 ml/min with a creatinine of 2.7, total volume of 1200 ml and 110 mg of proteinuria performed on March 1), most likely secondary to the following:
   a. Hypertension × 30+ years, inactivity problem.
   b. Postrenal causes, namely, bilateral hydronephrosis/bilateral UPJ obstruction, status post ureteral stent placement.
   c. Elderly age.
3. Asthma × 15 years. Continue Maxair and theophylline.
4. Gastroesophageal reflux disease. Continue Protonix.
5. Bilateral lower extremity edema, right more than the left secondary to chronic venous insufficiency/history of vein stripping, chronic renal failure (as noted above), and elderly age. Deep venous thrombosis has been ruled out by duplex ultrasound on admission.

At this time, I am going to sign off the case, and Dr. Avila will reassume care.

CPT Code(s): ____________________

ICD-10-CM Code(s): ____________________

ICD-9-CM Code(s): ____________________

Abstracting Questions

1. What type of service was provided? ____________________
2. Are both the acute and chronic renal failure diagnoses reported? ____________________
3. Does the chronic hypertension affect the renal failure diagnosis coding? ____________________

Case 8-2: Progress Note, Peritoneal Dialysis

LOCATION: Inpatient, Hospital

PATIENT: Betsy Morgon

ATTENDING PHYSICIAN: George Orbitz, MD

DATE OF SERVICE: Monday, April, 20XX. This patient had a good night. The dialysis for her end-stage renal disease went well. It dropped her weight less than a pound again as we had anticipated. Her diabetes is coming under good control with the 36 units of Glargine. Today we gave her 12 with breakfast. We discussed lunch. Will see how her glucose is before lunch. If it is less than 120, will back down to 10 units instead of 12 before lunch and do the same with supper. Will continue the same 2.5/1.5 peritoneal dialysis regimen tonight. So far the rehab progress has been excellent, dialysis has been going very well, and diabetes care is improved dramatically.

CPT Code(s): ____________________

ICD-10-CM Code(s): ____________________

ICD-9-CM Code(s): ____________________

Abstracting Questions

1. Was this encounter reported with an E/M code? ____________________
2. Does the type of dialysis affect the code selection? ____________________

Case 8-3: Progress Note, Cycler PD

LOCATION: Inpatient, Hospital

PATIENT: Sara Hildebrandt

ATTENDING PHYSICIAN: George Orbitz, MD

This patient with end-stage renal disease was reviewed. She is clinically stable. Her heart and lung exam is stable. Her weights were confusing this morning, but when we realized we did not factor in the full abdomen, which is probably at least 5 lb or more, and the titanium halo and collar, which were probably about 7 lb, we were probably pretty close. She came out on the scale at almost 183. If we subtract 12 lb for that, we are probably closer to 170 as a true weight. Her dry weight is probably around 158, so we are up some but not quite as much as the original scare weight would suggest. We are finishing the end of her cycler. We will eventually get a final drain weight and ultrafiltration rate, but my feeling at this time is that we will probably continue with the 2.5% Dianeal. We will put up another 18 liters, and we will put her on a cycle for 16 hours a day and leave her dry for about 8 hours a day so that she can participate in the physical therapy, and we will eventually shorten the cycler cycle.

The problem that we are dealing with is that whatever residual renal function she may have had will probably not be present anymore after all this surgery, so she will probably be better off with as much dialysis as she can get during times when she is not occupied with physical therapy activities. Eventually, we may even give her some daytime exchanges. Otherwise, she is doing well. We will use the same additives, and she will be able to transfer out of surgical ICU today.

She was re-examined several times during the morning, and she seems to be having no respiratory distress from the CAPD and the 2400 cc volume.

CPT Code(s): ______________________________

ICD-10-CM Code(s): ______________________________

ICD-9-CM Code(s): ______________________________

Abstracting Questions

1. What type of dialysis did the patient receive? ______________________________
2. The documentation indicates that the patient was "re-examined several times." Does this affect code selection?

   ____

Case 8-4: Renal Tumor Excision

LOCATION: Inpatient, Hospital

PATIENT: Brian Eberhoft

ATTENDING PHYSICIAN: Leslie Alanda, MD

SURGEON: Ira Avila, MD

PREOPERATIVE DIAGNOSIS: Right renal tumor.

POSTOPERATIVE DIAGNOSIS: Complex right renal cyst (acquired).

PROCEDURE PERFORMED: Right renal exploration; de-roofing of right renal cyst.

ANESTHESIA: General.

CLINICAL NOTE: Mr. Eberhoft is a 78-year-old gentleman found to have an enlarging right complex renal mass. This does not enhance but has irregular boundaries and has increased in size over the past year. It is located on the medial posterior part of the right kidney adjacent to the renal hilum. Options were discussed with the patient, and he elected to proceed with exploration and possible partial nephrectomy or radical nephrectomy depending on findings.

PROCEDURE: The patient was given a general endotracheal anesthetic as well as an epidural for intraoperative and postoperative analgesia. An incision was made over the tip of the 10th rib and the tip of the 10th rib excised. A small hole in the pleura was created, which was closed at the end of the case.

The patient has very poor fascial structures and very poor superficial muscle development. The peritoneal space was entered and the kidney identified. The Omni retractor was used for exposure. The ascending color was reflected off of Gerota's fascia. The duodenum had made a large turn over top of the renal hilum, and the duodenum was kocherized carefully. The renal vein and renal artery were identified, isolated, and surrounded with vessel loops.

The kidney was mobilized. The adrenal was quite superficial within Gerota's fascia, and the fascia was accidentally torn during the mobilization of the kidney. This was controlled with hemoclips. There was a large perinephric fat pad that was mobilized with the kidney initially, and then Gerota's fascia opened posteriorly. The area in question was identified. The patient had some reaction around the area, but this was not significant. There was a lot of fat adherent to the kidney that was dissected off the posterior region around the renal hilum to identify the mass. The mass appeared to be cystic in origin. A total of 3 cc of cyst fluid was aspirated from this and sent for cytology.

The cyst room was then opened. There was only a very small part of the cyst visible at the renal surface. Inspection of the cyst wall showed it to be smooth without masses. A small vessel was seen coursing inferiorly. This was cauterized. The renal pelvis was identified and Jelco catheter placed, and 5 cc of methylene blue–stained saline was injected through this to ensure that there was no communication with the cyst cavity and the renal pelvis. There was none.

The entire cyst wall was then cauterized. It was packed with Surgicel. Surgicel was also placed over the adrenal gland to help ensure hemostasis. Hemostasis was ensured. Vessel loops were removed. The kidney was then returned to renal fossa. A 10-mm Jackson-Pratt drain was left through a left lower quadrant stab wound and was placed adjacent to the de-roofed renal cyst.

The peritoneum was inspected, and there was no other abnormality identified on laparotomy.

The abdominal wall was then closed with three layers of 1 Vicryl. The skin was closed with surgical clips. A dressing was applied. Abdominal binder was applied. Prior to beginning closure of the abdominal wall, the rent in the pleura was closed with 3–0 Vicryl. Air was removed using a red rubber catheter in the usual fashion.

Sponge and needle counter were reported correct. The patient had a Foley catheter placed intraoperatively, and he had good urine output throughout the case. Estimated blood loss was 300 cc. He was transferred to the recovery room in good condition.

CPT Code(s): ________________________________

ICD-10-CM Code(s): ________________________________

ICD-9-CM Code(s): ________________________________

Abstracting Questions

1. Was this procedure reported as an excision, even though the cyst was drained and the cyst wall retained?

   ____
2. Was de-roofing of renal cyst the same as an excision? ________________________________
3. Did the accidental tear of the fascia require a separate, reportable repair? ________________________________
4. Was a modifier reported? ________________________________
5. Was the diagnosis for an acquired or congenital renal cyst? ________________________________

Case 8-5: Renal Mass

LOCATION: Inpatient, Hospital

PATIENT: Myra Grossman

ATTENDING PHYSICIAN: Ronald Green, MD

SURGEON: Ira Avila, MD

PREOPERATIVE DIAGNOSIS: Right renal mass.

POSTOPERATIVE DIAGNOSIS: Right renal cyst (acquired).

PROCEDURE PERFORMED: Laparoscopic exploration of kidneys, de-roofing, and biopsy of right renal mass.

ANESTHESIA: General.

SURGICAL INDICATIONS: This is a 20-year-old female who has a complex right renal cyst. She has been evaluated and worked up by Dr. Green. Options have been discussed, and she has elected to proceed with the exploration.

PROCEDURE: The patient was prepped and draped in the right flank position. A Foley catheter was placed. An incision was made. A retroperitoneal laparoscopic approach was used to approach the kidney, the cyst isolated, vessels identified and surrounded with vessel loops. The cyst was then aspirated and contents sent for cytology. The roof was ablated free and the base biopsied. There was some bleeding from the bases, which was controlled with 3–0 Chromic suture ligature. 3–0 Chromic sutures were used to close the cyst defect. A 10-mm flat Jackson-Pratt drain was left through a separate stab wound and sutured to the skin. The wound was closed with Vicryl and skin with clips. The patient tolerated the procedure well and was transferred to the recovery room in good condition. Estimated blood loss was 100 cc.

Pathology Report Later Indicated: Both pathology and cytology reports demonstrating benign cyst.

CPT Code(s): ____________________

ICD-10-CM Code(s): ____________________

ICD-9-CM Code(s): ____________________

Abstracting Questions

1. What surgical approach was used for this procedure? ____________________

Case 8-6: Renal Tumor

Code only Dr. Avila's services.

LOCATION: Inpatient, Hospital

PATIENT: Tommy Boyle

ATTENDING PHYSICIAN: Gary Sanchez, MD

SURGEON: Ira Avila, MD

PREOPERATIVE DIAGNOSIS: Left renal tumor.

POSTOPERATIVE DIAGNOSIS: Hemorrhagic cyst (acquired), left kidney.

PROCEDURE PERFORMED: Hemorrhagic cyst, left kidney, multiple renal biopsies. Incidental splenic laceration and splenectomy.

PROCEDURE: Please see previous notes for relevant past medical history. The patient did have an epidural, as well as general endotracheal anesthetic. Dr. Sanchez performed an AAA repair, and then I was asked to explore the kidney. The patient had significant adhesions of his greater mesentery and spleen to the left upper quadrant. Significant time was taken to mobilize this, and in doing so a small tear was made in the capsule of the spleen. Unfortunately at this point and because of the patient's prior anticoagulation, he was quite oozy. Prior to my beginning the dissection the hemoglobin came back at 5.3, therefore transfusion was begun. The patient remained stable for the most part during our dissection; however, his pressure did drop about 1 hour into the manipulation and was packed. The patient was transfused and his blood pressure stabilized. No other ECG changes or other abnormalities were noted.

The kidney was mobilized. Hemoclips were used to dissect off the adrenal gland superiorly. The lesion in question was identified in the upper pole of the kidney anteriorly. Fat was maintained over this lesion, and it was isolated. There was also a pale area on the lower pole of the kidney that was biopsied and found to be fibrotic, not representative of a tumor. Multiple biopsies from the lesion were taken, including the dome. Within the lesion was noted old hemorrhage; these were all sent for frozen section and found to be benign. No evidence of tumor was identified. It was thought that this likely represented a benign hemorrhagic cyst. Therefore, no further dissection was required.

Hemostasis was achieved with silk suture and Gelfoam. Unfortunately, the spleen continued to ooze, and it was believed in the patient's best interest that a splenectomy be performed by Dr. Sanchez and his team.

The wound was then closed by me using a #1 PDS. The skin was closed with surgical staples. The patient was transfused a total of six units of blood and two units of fresh frozen plasma. Sponge and needle counts were reported as correct. The patient was transferred to the surgical critical care unit in good condition.

Pathology Report Later Indicated: Benign tissue.

CPT Code(s): ______________________________

ICD-10-CM Code(s): ______________________________

ICD-9-CM Code(s): ______________________________

Abstracting Questions

1. There were significant adhesions that required significant time to mobilize. Would this process be reported separately? ______
2. Was a frozen section performed in addition to other biopsies? ______
3. Did the intraoperative frozen section results affect management of the renal cyst? ______
4. How was the tear in the splenic capsule treated? ______

Case 8-7: Dialysis Catheter Replacement

LOCATION: Outpatient, Hospital

PATIENT: Sally Perez

ATTENDING PHYSICIAN: George Orbitz, MD

SURGEON: George Orbitz, MD

PREOPERATIVE DIAGNOSIS: ESRD.

POSTOPERATIVE DIAGNOSIS: ESRD.

PROCEDURE PERFORMED: Dialysis catheter replacement.

ANESTHESIA: Local.

DESCRIPTION OF PROCEDURE: After obtaining consent, the 46-year-old patient was put in the Trendelenburg position. The area of the right IJ vein where the catheter was placed was prepped in the usual fashion. A guidewire was advanced without difficulty. The old dialysis catheter was taken out. Tip was sent for culture. A new 11.5 French 13.5-cm temporary dialysis catheter was advanced through the right IJ vein over the guidewire using the Seldinger technique without difficulty. Both ports had good blood return. Both ports were flushed with saline and heparin. The catheter was secured to the skin. The patient tolerated the procedure well without immediate complications.

CPT Code(s): ____________________

ICD-10-CM Code(s): ____________________

ICD-9-CM Code(s): ____________________

Abstracting Questions

1. Was the catheter placement venous or arterial? ____________________
2. Was this an open or percutaneous insertion? ____________________
3. Was the catheter a central or peripheral insertion? ____________________
4. Was this reported as an insertion or a replacement? ____________________
5. What was the principal reason for the encounter? ____________________

Chapter 9

Neurology and Ophthalmology

Case 9-1: Intracerebral Hematoma

OPERATIVE PROCEDURE

LOCATION: Inpatient, Hospital

PATIENT: Suzy Kunklemann

ATTENDING PHYSICIAN: Gary Sanchez, MD

SURGEON: Gary Sanchez, MD

PREOPERATIVE DIAGNOSIS: Intracerebral hematoma (nontraumatic), right temporal lobe.

POSTOPERATIVE DIAGNOSIS: Intracerebral hematoma (nontraumatic), right temporal lobe.

PROCEDURE PERFORMED: Osteoplastic craniotomy, right temporal area; evacuation of intracerebral hematoma.

ANESTHESIA: General.

PROCEDURE: Under general anesthesia, the patient's head was placed in the Mayfield pins. The right frontal temporoparietal area was prepped and draped in the usual manner. A linear incision was made extending from the midline of the temporal fossa up to the midportion of the scalp. The skin was incised. The temporalis muscle was separated and divided off the bone. I did a craniotomy here the size of a half-dollar and made a burr hole. I utilized the craniotome to elevate the bone flap, and this was a free bone flap. This was then removed. We placed the Weitlaners into the wound and then incised the dura in a cruciate fashion over the temporal lobe. I then entered the middle temple gyrus and irrigated much of the clot from the temporal and posterior parietal areas, and evacuated the clot from the area. This took copious irrigation. We used cotton balls for hemostasis. I did this numerous times until all the bleeders were coagulated. I then lined the cystic cavity with Gelfoam and coagulated the edges of the raw brain. I closed the dura with 4–0 Vicryl. This was closed in a watertight fashion. I used 2–0 Vicryl to elevate the dura to the bone flap with Wurzburg plates, two of them, utilizing plates and screws. I then closed the scalp in one layer using 0 Vicryl on the temporalis muscle and fascia, and the skin was approximated with 2–0 nylon interrupted mattress sutures. Dressing was applied, and the patient was on the ventilator and discharged to the surgical intensive care unit.

CPT Code(s): ________________________________

ICD-10-CM Code(s): ________________________________

ICD-9-CM Code(s): ________________________________

Abstracting Questions

1. Was the procedure performed a surgical craniotomy? ________________________________
2. Does the area of the skull being opened affect the code? ________________________________
3. What was the purpose of the procedure? ________________________________
4. Does the purpose of the procedure affect the CPT code? ________________________________

Case 9-2: Release of Ulnar Nerve and Cubital Tunnel

OPERATIVE PROCEDURE

LOCATION: Outpatient, Hospital

PATIENT: Brian Orwell

ATTENDING PHYSICIAN: Gary Sanchez, MD

SURGEON: Gary Sanchez, MD

PREOPERATIVE DIAGNOSIS: Tardive ulnar nerve palsy, left.

POSTOPERATIVE DIAGNOSIS: Tardive ulnar nerve palsy, left.

PROCEDURE PERFORMED: Release of ulnar nerve and cubital tunnel.

ANESTHESIA: General.

PROCEDURE: A curvilinear incision was made over the cubital tunnel. The dissection was taken down to the cubital tunnel. The nerve was localized. It was freed up in the tunnel up to where it enters the flexor carpi ulnaris. Fat was oversewn with 2–0 chromic. The wound was approximated with 2–0 plain, and the subcuticular tissue with 4–0 nylon interrupted mattress sutures in the skin.

CPT Code(s): ______________________________

ICD-10-CM Code(s): ______________________________

ICD-9-CM Code(s): ______________________________

Abstracting Questions

1. Was the approach at the wrist or the elbow? ______________________________
2. What is the term for "nerve release"? ______________________________
3. Does the term "tardive" (meaning "late") affect diagnosis code selection for the ulnar nerve palsy?

   ____

Case 9-3: Parietal Burr Holes

OPERATIVE PROCEDURE

LOCATION: Inpatient, Hospital

PATIENT: Reed Scaleni

ATTENDING PHYSICIAN: Gary Sanchez, MD

SURGEON: Gary Sanchez, MD

PREOPERATIVE DIAGNOSIS: Subacute subdural hematoma (nontraumatic), right side.

POSTOPERATIVE DIAGNOSIS: Subacute subdural hematoma (nontraumatic), right side.

PROCEDURE PERFORMED: Burr hole times two, right frontal and right posterior parietal.

ANESTHESIA: General.

PROCEDURE: Under general anesthesia, the patient's head was prepped and draped in the usual manner. The incision was made. Straight line linear incisions over the frontal and posterior parietal areas were made on the right side. Retractors were placed. Burr holes remained. The dura was visualized. The bony edges were waxed with beeswax. The dura was incised, both the frontal and the parietal holes. Serosanguineous fluid and clouded blood exuded. I cleaned it out until the supernatant was clear. The brain was found to be pulsating beneath. We then placed two medium-size Penrose drains and closed the galea with 2–0 Vicryl. The skin was approximated with surgical staples, and the Penrose drains were anchored with sutures. A dressing was applied. The patient was discharged to the PAR.

CPT Code(s): ____________________

ICD-10-CM Code(s): ____________________

ICD-9-CM Code(s): ____________________

Abstracting Questions

1. What determines the code assignment for burr holes of the skull? ____________________
2. Does the location of the hematoma being drained/aspirated make a difference in the CPT code assignment? ____________________
3. Was this CPT code reported twice for the two burr holes? ____________________
4. Was a modifier reported to indicate which side of the skull was drilled? ____________________

Case 9-4: Discectomy

OPERATIVE PROCEDURE

LOCATION: Inpatient, Hospital

PATIENT: Muriel Limbaugh

ATTENDING PHYSICIAN: Gary Sanchez, MD

SURGEON: Gary Sanchez, MD

PREOPERATIVE DIAGNOSIS: Right L4-5 and L5-S1 herniated disc.

POSTOPERATIVE DIAGNOSIS: Right L4-5 and L5-S1 herniated disc.

OPERATIVE PROCEDURE
1. Right L4-5 discectomy.
2. Right L5-S1 discectomy.

INDICATION: This is a 21-year-old female who presented with a greater than 1-year history of right leg pain. It was refractory to conservative treatment. MRI scan showed a severely bulging L4-5 and L5-S1 discs on the right. After a discussion of the options, she elected surgery. The risks were thoroughly discussed, and the patient gave her consent.

PROCEDURE: The patient was taken to the operating room and underwent induction of general endotracheal anesthesia in the supine position. The patient was then flipped to the prone position on the operating room table. The hips and the knees were flexed. The lumbosacral area was thoroughly prepped and draped, and a vertical midline skin incision was made over the L4-5 and S1 spinous processes after the skin was infiltrated with local anesthetic. Using the monopolar cautery, I dissected through the subcutaneous tissue in the midline down to the spinous processes of L4-5 and S1. I then used the periosteal elevator and retracted the paraspinal muscles laterally along L4-5 and S1. An intraoperative x-ray was then taken, which verified that the marker was at the L4-5 interspace. I then removed the inferior 4 mm of the lamina of L4 with a Kerrison rongeur. I then incised the ligamentum flavum with a #15 blade down to the epidural fat. I retracted the common dural sac and the right L5 nerve root medially. I palpated a very significant bulge underneath the root. I then incised the annulus and removed several pieces of disc, which were bulging into the spinal canal. I then took a nerve hook and placed it underneath the dural space adjacent to the disc space and depressed the bulging disc space into the cavity I had created. I then removed additional pieces of disc. I then explored with a nerve hook and was content that the dural sac and the right L5 nerve root were nicely decompressed. Hemostasis was achieved with a bipolar cautery and strategically placed pieces of Surgicel. I irrigated with saline. An epidural fat graft was placed. I then reoriented my retractor toward the L5-S1 interspace. I removed the inferior 3 mm of the lamina of L5 with the Kerrison rongeur. I then incised the ligamentum flavum and resected it with the Kerrison rongeurs. I then retracted the common dural sac and the right S1 nerve root medially. There was a definite bulge within the disc space but not as significant as the above level. I incised the disc and removed additional pieces. I then decompressed the bulging annulus into the cavity I had created and removed additional disc. I was content after exploration with a nerve hook that the dural sac and S1 nerve root was nicely decompressed on the right. I then irrigated with copious amounts of saline. An epidural fat graft was placed. The wound was closed in layers with interrupted 0 and 2–0 Vicryl. The skin was closed with a running 3–0 Vicryl subcuticular stitch. Benzoin, Steri-Strips, and a sterile dressing were placed.

The patient tolerated the procedure well without apparent complication. Sponge, instrument, and needle counts were correct. The patient was taken to the recovery room after the surgery.

CPT Code(s): ______________________________

ICD-10-CM Code(s): ______________________________

ICD-9-CM Code(s): ______________________________

Abstracting Questions

1. In addition to the discectomy, what other procedure was performed that affects code assignment?

   ____

2. Was the procedure approach anterior or posterior? ______________________________
3. What are the two levels of the spine referenced in the medical report? ______________________________
4. Upon what two disc spaces did the surgeon perform discectomies? ______________________________
5. How many CPT codes were required to report the disc repairs? ______________________________
6. What modifier was reported on the CPT codes? ______________________________

Case 9-5: Carpal Tunnel

OPERATIVE PROCEDURE

LOCATION: Outpatient, Hospital

PATIENT: Judy Burns

ATTENDING PHYSICIAN: Gary Sanchez, MD

SURGEON: Gary Sanchez, MD

PREOPERATIVE DIAGNOSIS: Left carpal tunnel syndrome.

POSTOPERATIVE DIAGNOSIS: Left carpal tunnel syndrome.

PROCEDURE PERFORMED: Carpal tunnel released, left wrist.

ANESTHESIA: Regional.

PROCEDURE: After a satisfactory level of regional anesthesia, the extremity was addressed once it had been sterilely prepped and draped. Throughout the procedure the patient needed some focal augmentation for sharp pain characteristics at the level of the skin most distally about the skin wound. Sharp dissection was conducted down to the palmaris fascia. We identified the deep transverse ligament. In a blunt manner, we undermined this, and with use of a Freer interposing between deep transverse carpal ligament and the medial nerve, sharply dissected over the Freer, releasing the impinging structures about the carpal canal. The probe palpation, the tendinous structures, and the floor of the carpal canal were otherwise unremarkable. She has at this time an exiting thenar motor branch, which was not obscured. There is an hourglass deformity of the median nerve as noted. At completion of this the wound was irrigated, followed by closure of the dermal planes and application of a splint. The patient tolerated the procedure well and was transported to the recovery room in a stable manner.

CPT Code(s): ______________________________

ICD-10-CM Code(s): ______________________________

ICD-9-CM Code(s): ______________________________

Abstracting Questions

1. Release of the carpal tunnel has what effect on the median nerve? ______________________________

Case 9-6: Repair of Pseudomeningocele

OPERATIVE PROCEDURE

This patient is returned to the operating room during the postoperative period for a decompression laminectomy performed by the same physician who now performs the pseudomeningocele repair.

LOCATION: Inpatient, Hospital

PATIENT: Debbie Smith

ATTENDING PHYSICIAN: Gary Sanchez, MD

SURGEON: Gary Sanchez, MD

PREOPERATIVE DIAGNOSIS: Pseudomeningocele.

POSTOPERATIVE DIAGNOSIS: Pseudomeningocele.

PROCEDURE PERFORMED: Repair of pseudomeningocele at the L4-5 level just to the left of the midline.

PROCEDURE: The patient was taken to the operating room and underwent placement of a spinal drain by the anesthesiologist. She then underwent induction of a general endotracheal anesthesia. She was flipped to the prone position and was thoroughly prepped and draped. The previous incision was reopened and was extended approximately 1 inch both superiorly and inferiorly. A large amount of spinal fluid came forth. There was a well-epithelialized membrane underneath the subcutaneous tissue extending deep to the muscle. This was excised as much as possible. I first dissected the paraspinal muscles laterally on each side along the L2 vertebra. I identified epithelial lining consistent with a pseudomeningocele. I saw a small leak and thought that I saw spinal fluid coming from the small defect. I gave a Valsalva maneuver, but it was not crystal clear whether this was spinal fluid or merely epidural blood. Anyway, I packed this off with Surgicel, placed a small fat graft, and secured it with a 4–0 Nurolon. I then used the FloSeal and Duragen to seal off the defect. I began reapproximating the muscle when I then noticed that there was spinal fluid again coming from the inferior portion of the incision. I exposed the lamina of L5 bilaterally and placed a retractor. I then noticed that there was a dural defect just to the left of the midline between the L4 and L5 laminae. I did a partial hemilaminectomy of L5 on the left side and was able to place three separate 4–0 Nurolon sutures through the dural defect. Care was taken to depress the nerve within the dural sac with a #4 Penfield. I then directly repaired the dura and did not see any further spinal fluid leakage with a Valsalva maneuver. I then used some FloSeal and strategically placed pieces of Surgicel to cover the defect. I then placed a small piece of Duragen on top of this as well. I irrigated with copious amounts of saline. I then closed the muscle in the deep fascia with interrupted 2–0 Vicryls, which were very closely approximated. I then used interrupted 2–0 Vicryl to close the subcutaneous tissue. The skin was closed with a running 4–0 nylon interlocking stitch. A sterile dressing was placed.

The patient tolerated the procedure well without apparent complications. The spinal drain was sutured in by me at the end of the procedure. She was taken to the recovery room in stable condition. Sponge, instrument, and needle counts were correct times two.

CPT Code(s): ______________________________

ICD-10-CM Code(s): ______________________________

ICD-9-CM Code(s): ______________________________

Abstracting Questions

1. Repair of the pseudomeningocele is repair of what? ____________________
2. What procedure was performed to clear the approach for the repair of the dura tear? ____________________
3. Does the pseudomeningocele make a difference in the CPT code assignment? ____________________
4. What modifiers are required? ____________________

Case 9-7: Laminectomy with Foraminotomy

OPERATIVE PROCEDURE

LOCATION: Inpatient, Hospital

PATIENT: Karen Origami

ATTENDING PHYSICIAN: Gary Sanchez, MD

SURGEON: Gary Sanchez, MD

PREOPERATIVE DIAGNOSIS: Severe spinal stenosis from L3 through L5.

POSTOPERATIVE DIAGNOSIS: Severe spinal stenosis from L3 through L5 without neurogenic claudications.

PROCEDURES PERFORMED
1. Bilateral L3 laminectomy with foraminotomy.
2. Bilateral L4 laminectomy with foraminotomy.
3. Bilateral L5 laminectomy with foraminotomy.

INDICATION: This patient is a 79-year-old female who presented with severe neurogenic claudication, left greater than right. Workup included an MRI scan, which showed severe spinal stenosis from L3 through L5. After discussion of the options, she elected to undergo surgery. She was informed that this was an elective surgery and was not life or limb threatening. The risks of the procedure were thoroughly discussed, and the patient consented to proceed.

PROCEDURE: The patient was taken to the operating room and underwent induction after general endotracheal anesthesia in the supine position. She was then flipped to the prone position on the operating room table and the knees were flexed. The lower lumbar spine was thoroughly prepped and draped, and a vertical midline skin incision was made from the L3 to the S1 spinous processes. The skin was infiltrated with local anesthetic prior to making the incision. Using the monopolar cautery, I identified the spinous processes of L2 through S1 bilaterally. Then using the periosteal elevator, I retracted the paraspinal muscles laterally bilaterally. Deep retractors were placed. At this point, I used the handheld rongeur and removed the spinous processes of L4 and L3. An intraoperative x-ray was done to verify the location. At this, the L5 spinous process was then removed. I then alternated between the rongeurs and the high-speed burr, and drilled down the medial facets and the lamina of L5, L4, and L3. I then began using the Kerrison and removed the inferior lamina of L5 and proceeded from a caudal to cephalad direction. I alternated between the high-speed drill and the Kerrison rongeurs and eventually removed the lamina and the medial facets bilaterally of L3 through L5. There was noted to be very severe compression of the thecal sac at the L4-5 level as there was a grade 1 spondylolisthesis at that level. There was also noted to be severe spinal stenosis at the L3-4 level. After an adequate decompression, I made sure that the decompression extended laterally out to the exiting nerve roots on each side bilaterally. The nerve roots were particularly tight at the L4-5 level, where the spondylolisthesis was located. At no time was there a dural tear or spinal fluid leak. I irrigated with copious amounts of saline. Bleeding bone edges were waxed. The gutters were lined with Surgicel, and a piece of Gelfoam was placed over the exposed dura. I irrigated again. I closed the wound in layers with interrupted 0 and 2–0 Vicryl. Skin was closed with a running 3–0 Vicryl subcuticular stitch. Benzoin and one-half-inch Steri-Strips and a sterile dressing were placed.

The patient tolerated the procedure well without apparent complication. She will go to the recovery room after the surgery. Sponge, instrument, and needle counts were correct.

CPT Code(s): ________________________________

ICD-10-CM Code(s): ________________________________

ICD-9-CM Code(s): ________________________________

Abstracting Questions

1. In addition to the laminectomy with foraminotomy, what other procedure was performed? ____________
2. Which vertebrae were addressed? ________________________________
3. How many codes are necessary to report all three vertebrae? ____________________
4. What modifiers are required? ________________________________

Case 9-8: Laminotomy, Discectomy, and Foraminotomy

Report the monitoring with sensory-evoked potentials.

LOCATION: Inpatient, Hospital

PATIENT: David Williams

ATTENDING PHYSICIAN: Timothy Pleasant, MD

SURGEON: Timothy Pleasant, MD

PREOPERATIVE DIAGNOSIS: Spondylolisthesis L5-S1 (acquired), recurrent disc L5-S1.

POSTOPERATIVE DIAGNOSIS: Spondylolisthesis grade 1, L5-S1. Disc L5-S1.

PROCEDURES PERFORMED
1. Pedicle screws L5 to sacrum.
2. Decompressive laminotomy and foraminotomy on the left at L5-S1.
3. Removal of disc at L5-S1.
4. Taking of homograft from right hip.
5. Transverse body fusion L5 to sacrum.
6. Placement of Dyna-Lok system on pedicle screws with distraction of L5-S1.

ANESTHESIA: General.

Prior to the surgery this patient has been counseled regarding the expectations of said surgery, the possibility of complications, infection, weakness in the leg, persistent numbness, possibility of dural tear because of the adhesions, and the possibility of not being able to relieve his pain. The patient understands all of this and is willing to undergo surgery.

This surgery was done with Stealth navigator and utilizing Stealth for placement of pedicle screws. The patient was also monitored throughout the case with sensory-evoked potentials.

PROCEDURE: Under general anesthesia the patient was placed in the prone position; the back was prepped and draped in the usual manner. The previous incision was incised. We exposed the spinous processes of L3-L4, L5, and the sacrum. The erector spini muscles were taken down so as to expose the pedicle and transverse process on the right side, as well as on the left side. The pedicles of L5-S1 and L4-5 were localized. Debrided the transverse process to sacrum of all tissues in preparation for the graft.

The procedure continued in the following manner. We placed, under Stealth navigation, the pedicle screw down the pedicle of L5 and then placed a screw down the ala of the sacrum. These were braced utilizing Stealth protocol by using the awl, the probe, and verifying the distance of screw and placement of screw with Stealth. This was done on the right side first, and then we proceeded to do it on the left side. The screws having been placed, attention was directed to the left side, where we increased the laminotomy and freed up the L5 root by increasing the foraminotomy and the S1 root. We saw the softened disc here and entered the disc space and removed degenerating material. The disc was decompressed on the way out with one of the pituitaries, and I think we took a strand of one of the dorsal roots. This was only one strand and was sent for specimen. There was no dural leak. I think this came from the underside of the L5 root. There was a multitude of adhesions there. The L5 root appeared very swollen, reddened, and the dura was very thinned out. Having decompressed the roots, we were satisfied with the decompression and now paid attention to taking the homograft with the reamer from the right hip by incising the gluteal fascia. We utilized the reamer on two passes to gain access to cortical cancellous bone. The graft sites had been prepared with the burr. We roughed up and denuded the bony surfaces, both transverse process and the ala, plus the L5-S1 area. Having done this, I then was satisfied that I had enough graft from the spinous processes of the laminotomy we had done, plus the donor site, plus we utilized cortical cancellous homograft. We then placed our Dyna-Lok system onto the screws and produced distraction of a few mm, perhaps 3, on the screws between L5 and S1. We then secured these screws and the system tightly to 120 pounds of pressure. The wound was then irrigated. A fat graft was placed over the laminotomy site. The bone graft was then mixed with the homograft and allograft and placed on the transverse processes and the lamina; we used osteoblast glue as well. We also used osteoblast glue to place on the donor sites with the graft. I then closed the wound in layers using double-knotted 0 chromic on the lumbodorsal fascia, 0 Vicryl on the subcutaneous tissue, and 2–0 plain on the subcuticular tissue and surgical staples on the skin. The gluteus fascia was also approximated with 0 Vicryl, and beeswax was placed on the bony denuded surfaces. A dressing was placed. The patient was discharged to the recovery room.

OPERATION PERFORMED
1. Redo laminotomy, foraminotomy, and discectomy at L5-S1 on the left.
2. Placement of pedicle screws L5 in the sacrum with Dyna-Lok system that is an arthrodesis.
3. Taking of homograft from the right hip.
4. Transverse and laminar fusion.

To be noted, the case was complicated by minor dural tear on the undersurface of the root. No repair was required, except placing a fat graft on top of the dura. No CSF leak was visualized.

CPT Code(s): ____________________

ICD-10-CM Code(s): ____________________

ICD-9-CM Code(s): ____________________

Abstracting Questions

1. What vertebra had the laminotomy/foraminotomy? ____________________
2. How was this procedure identified as a re-exploration? ____________________
3. Discectomy was performed for what level(s)? ____________________
4. Was the discectomy separately reported? ____________________
5. At what level(s) was there fusion performed? ____________________
6. What type of graft was used for the fusion? ____________________
7. What type of instrumentation was used? ____________________
8. What CPT code reports the computer-assisted stereotaxis? ____________________
9. What CPT code reports the evoked potentials? ____________________

Case 9-9: Halo Crown and Vest

Report the external cause code/E code for this injury.

LOCATION: Inpatient, Hospital

PATIENT: Billy Norton

ATTENDING PHYSICIAN: Timothy Pleasant, MD

SURGEON: Timothy Pleasant, MD

PREOPERATIVE DIAGNOSIS: Neck injury, motor vehicle accident.

POSTOPERATIVE DIAGNOSIS: Same as Preoperative.

PROCEDURE PERFORMED: Placement of halo crown and vest.

ANESTHESIA: Local.

SURGICAL INDICATIONS: This 62-year-old patient was in a motor vehicle accident and appears to have sustained a spinal cord injury with ligamentous instability at C4-5. He could not be placed in a neck collar because he has a short, thick neck and also because he had a tracheostomy tube. The patient would not be stabilized with traction as he has a distraction injury. It was indicated to place him in a halo vest and crown to immobilize his neck.

PROCEDURE: The hair was shaved behind both ears. There was a sterile prep done along the forehead region and the region behind both ears. The halo crown was then positioned and stabilized with the three positioners anteriorly and two laterally. I then injected Xylocaine behind both ears and along the supraorbital ridge laterally. I then placed the four pins and torqued them to 8 pounds per sq inch. The hexagonal lock nuts were then tightened. The patient tolerated this well without any apparent complications. The halo vest was then connected to the crown. The crown was placed. A large vest was used, but this was still too small for the patient, and on the right side the vest had to be tied with string until some permanent straps could be fashioned by orthotics. During the placement of the vest, I maintained the neck in neutral position and at no time was there any rotation or flexion or extension of the neck.

CPT Code(s): ______________________________

ICD-10-CM Code(s): ______________________________

ICD-9-CM Code(s): ______________________________

Abstracting Questions

1. What factor determines the code reported for placement of the halo? ______________________________
2. What factor influences fifth-digit assignment of the ICD-9-CM diagnosis code for the spinal cord injury?

   ____
3. Should an external cause/E code be reported? ______________________________

Case 9-10: Extracapsular Cataract

OPERATIVE PROCEDURE

LOCATION: Outpatient, Hospital

PATIENT: Carol Cassanda

ATTENDING PHYSICIAN: Rita Wimer, MD

SURGEON: Rita Wimer, MD

PREOPERATIVE DIAGNOSIS: Senile posterior subcapsular cataract—diffuse (with advancement on visual inspection compared with office visit), right eye.

POSTOPERATIVE DIAGNOSIS: Same as Preoperative.

PROCEDURE PERFORMED: Cataract extraction by phacoemulsification, right eye.

COMPLICATIONS: None.

ESTIMATED BLOOD LOSS: Minimal.

PROCEDURE: In the operating room a drop of lidocaine 4%-MPF was applied to the eye. The patient was prepped and draped in the usual sterile fashion for an intraocular procedure of the right eye. A lid speculum was placed. A Weck-cel soaked with lidocaine 4%-MPF was placed at the limbus in the area of the planned phaco side-port incision. A keratome was used to enter the chamber at the arcade. A small amount of preservative-free 1% lidocaine was injected into the anterior chamber. The aqueous was exchanged with viscoelastic material, and a side-port incision was made with a 15-degree angle blade. A continuous tear capsulotomy was made with a bent needle and the Utrata forceps. The nucleus was hydrodissected. Phacoemulsification was used to remove the nucleus using an ultrasound time of 2 minutes and 2 seconds and a phaco percentage of 3.92%. Irrigation and aspiration were used to remove the remaining cortical material. There was a pinhead-size piece of cortex, which appeared to be posterior to the capsule. There was no sign of an opening in the capsule, but it is possible that there was some peripheral zonule dehiscence, which could have allowed this to occur. In any case, it was small and it is expected to absorb without sequelae, and there was no sign of vitreous prolapse. The capsule was polished and vacuumed as indicated. A small additional amount of nonpreserved 1% lidocaine was again injected into the anterior chamber. The chamber was deepened with viscoelastic, and the posterior chamber intraocular lens was injected into the capsule bag and dialed into position. The remaining viscoelastic material was removed with irrigation and aspiration. The globe was pressurized and the cornea was hydrated to ensure a good seal. The wound was tested and found to be watertight. TobraDex drops were placed on the surface of the eye.

The patient left the operating room in stable condition without complications, having tolerated the procedure well.

CPT Code(s): ______________________________

ICD-10-CM Code(s): ______________________________

ICD-9-CM Code(s): ______________________________

Abstracting Questions

1. Does the intracapsular aspect affect the CPT code assignment for the cataract removal? ______
2. Is the replacement of the lens separately reported? ______
3. What terms in the cataract code description affected diagnosis coding? ______

Chapter 10
Obstetrics and Gynecology

Case 10-1: Abdominal Hysterectomy

OPERATIVE REPORT

LOCATION: Inpatient, Hospital

PATIENT: Maggie Brock

ATTENDING PHYSICIAN: Andy Martinez, MD

SURGEON: Andy Martinez, MD

PREOPERATIVE DIAGNOSES
1. Chronic menorrhagia.
2. Uterine fibroids.

POSTOPERATIVE DIAGNOSES
1. Chronic menorrhagia.
2. Uterine fibroids.

PROCEDURE PERFORMED: Total abdominal hysterectomy and bilateral salpingo-oophorectomy.

ANESTHESIA: General endotracheal.

SURGICAL INDICATION: This patient is a 48-year-old multiparous female who had had problems with chronic menorrhagia, unsuccessfully treated with hormone manipulation. She had known fibroids as well. Endometrial biopsy preoperatively was benign.

OPERATIVE FINDINGS: The uterus was about 10- to 12-week size with multiple leiomyomas. There was a functional-appearing cyst on the left ovary that contained some clear fluid. The right ovary was normal. The appendix was retrocecal but otherwise unremarkable.

OPERATIVE DESCRIPTION: After induction of general anesthesia, the patient was in the supine position. The abdomen and vagina were prepped, and Foley catheter placed; the patient was then draped. The abdomen was opened through a midline hypogastric incision, excising the old skin scar on the way in. Bowel was then packed out of the pelvis and a self-retaining Balfour retractor was placed. The uterus was elevated with clamps at the cornual areas. The left round ligament was clamped, divided, suture ligated with 0 Vicryl. All sutures were 0 Vicryl unless otherwise indicated. The peritoneal lateral to the left infundibulopelvic ligament was opened with Metzenbaum scissors, isolated in the left ovarian vasculature. This pedicle was isolated, clamped, divided, and doubly ligated. An identical procedure was carried out in the structures on the right side. The anterior and posterior leaves of the broad ligament were taken down with Metzenbaum scissors. There was some abnormal scarring and retraction of the bladder flap on the left side due to her prior cesarean sections. We then skeletonized the uterine artery pedicles on either side. The uterine artery pedicles were clamped with curved Rogers clamps, cut, and suture ligated. The cardinal ligaments and paracervical tissue were taken with two bites of straight Heaney-Ballantine clamps and suture ligated. The vaginal angle was then clamped with curved Rogers clamps, cut and held. The anterior vagina was opened with scalpel; then the upper vagina was incised circumferentially with right-angled scissors. The uterus was then removed and handed off. The vaginal angles were sutured with 0 Vicryl, and the vaginal cuff was closed with a series of interrupted figure-of-eight 0 Vicryl sutures. There was a small bleeding area on one of the cardinal ligament pedicles on the left side. This was isolated with an Allis clamp and secured with a suture ligature. Sponges were then removed. Sponge and needle counts were correct. The abdominal fascia was closed with interrupted 0 Ethibond sutures and the skin with staples. Blood loss estimation by anesthesia was 250 cc. Specimen to pathology: Uterus, tubes, and ovaries. Final sponge and needle counts were correct.

CPT Code(s): ______________________________

ICD-10-CM Code(s): ______________________________

ICD-9-CM Code(s): ______________________________

Abstracting Questions

1. What factors affect CPT code assignment for the abdominal hysterectomy? ______________________________
2. What factors affect the diagnosis code selection for the uterine leiomyoma? ______________________________
3. What is another name for leiomyoma? ______________________________

Case 10-2: Dilation and Curettage

OPERATIVE REPORT

LOCATION: Inpatient, Hospital

PATIENT: Sandy Porter

PRIMARY CARE PHYSICIAN: Andy Martinez, MD

SURGEON: Andy Martinez, MD

PREOPERATIVE DIAGNOSIS: Dysfunctional uterine bleeding.

POSTOPERATIVE DIAGNOSIS: Dysfunctional uterine bleeding.

PROCEDURE PERFORMED: Dilation and curettage of the uterus and diagnostic hysteroscopy.

SURGICAL INDICATIONS: This patient is a 38-year-old female whose last delivery was a little over a year ago. She started having periods every 2 weeks over the past few months. She had recently had what was thought to be a false-positive serum HCG level at greater than 91,000. A urine HCG was negative, and a second sample sent to the Paradise Valley Clinic was negative. She had an ultrasound, which showed slight irregularity in the uterine cavity.

OPERATIVE FINDINGS: The uterus is 8.5 cm deep. There was a very slight irregularity along the posterior aspect of the endometrial cavity; however, this was possibly just due to grooving from the dilation process. No definite polyps were noted. The tubal ostia were both seen easily.

OPERATIVE DESCRIPTION: After induction of spinal anesthesia, the patient was placed in the dorsal lithotomy position. The perineum and vagina were prepped, bladder straight catheterized, and the patient draped. Bimanual exam was carried out and uterus was anterior and normal size. Adnexa revealed no masses. A weighted speculum was placed in the vagina and the cervix grasped with a single-tooth tenaculum. The endocervical canal was dilated to 7 mm with Hegar dilators. The 5.5-mm Olympus hysteroscope was introduced using normal saline as the distention medium. Photographs were taken of the endometrial cavity. The hysteroscope was withdrawn, and the sharp endometrial curettage was done. Hysteroscope was reinserted and no sign of perforation was seen. The endometrium looked fragmented.

Blood loss estimation was 5 cc. Specimen to pathology: Endometrial curettings. The patient tolerated the procedure well except for an incident during the prep when some of the Betadine prep solution apparently splashed up into the patient's eye. This was washed out by anesthesia.

CPT Code(s): ______________________________

ICD-10-CM Code(s): ______________________________

ICD-9-CM Code(s): ______________________________

Abstracting Questions

1. What factor affected the code assignment of the D&C? ______________________________
2. Was the hysteroscopy therapeutic or diagnostic? ______________________________

Case 10-3: Cesarean Section

OPERATIVE REPORT

The physician who performs the cesarean section will also provide the postpartum care in this case.

LOCATION: Inpatient, Hospital

PATIENT: Joan Tisdale

ATTENDING PHYSICIAN: Andy Martinez, MD

SURGEON: Andy Martinez, MD

PREOPERATIVE DIAGNOSES
1. Intrauterine pregnancy at 31 weeks and 6 days.
2. Abruptio placentae.

POSTOPERATIVE DIAGNOSES
1. Intrauterine pregnancy at 31 weeks and 6 days.
2. Abruptio placentae.

PROCEDURE PERFORMED: Primary low transverse cervical cesarean section.

ANESTHESIA: General endotracheal.

SURGICAL INDICATIONS: The patient is a 31-year-old woman, gravida 4, para 3, at 31 weeks 6 days by menstrual dates, who was transferred on an emergency basis because of uterine bleeding. She had an apparent abruption on ultrasound, and the vagina was filled with blood clot. For these reasons, she was taken to surgery for an emergency cesarean section.

OPERATIVE FINDINGS: The infant is female, born at 2007 hours, weighing 2125 grams (4 lb 10 ounces), with Apgar scores of 8 at 1 minute and 9 at 5 minutes. There was a lot of blood in the uterine cavity and some adherent clot to the placenta, estimated to be less than 10% abruption. The tubes and ovaries were normal.

PROCEDURE: The abdomen was prepped and draped. A Foley catheter was in. The patient was then given a general endotracheal anesthetic, and the abdomen was opened through a Pfannenstiel incision. Bladder flap was opened transversely with scissors, and bladder was dissected downward bluntly with a hand. A small incision was made in the myometrium of the lower uterine segment, and then entry into the uterus was accomplished bluntly with a Kelly clamp. Low transverse incision was made with bandage scissors. The infant was delivered without undue difficulty. The infant's mouth and nose were suctioned with a bulb syringe, the cord was clamped and cut, and the infant was handed to Dr. Ortez and the ICN staff. A segment of the cord was taken for cord blood gases, and the placenta was then delivered manually. Inspection of the uterine incision revealed there was a brisk bleeder near the left corner of the incision, and this was oversewn initially and the first layer was a running locked 0 Vicryl. The second layer was a running horizontal Lembert 0 Vicryl. The pelvis was irrigated with saline. The uterine incision was inspected, and there was a small amount of oozing from the incision, which was controlled with a single figure-of-eight 0 Vicryl suture. When hemostasis was adequate and lap sponges were correct, attention was directed toward closure. The peritoneum was loosely approximated in the midline with a couple of mattress sutures of 2–0 Vicryl. A medium Hemovac drain was placed subfascially to exit below the right side of the incision. The fascia was closed with running 0 Vicryl using two strands, one from either side to the middle and tied independently. The skin was closed with staples and the drain sutured to the skin with silk. Estimated blood loss was 1200-1500 cc.

Specimen to pathology was placenta. Final sponge and needle counts were correct.

CPT Code(s): ______________________________

ICD-10-CM Code(s): ______________________________

ICD-9-CM Code(s): ______________________________

Abstracting Questions

1. What factor in this case determines the appropriate c-section code? ______________________________
2. In addition to the placental abruption, what other two diagnoses must be reported? ________________ and ________________

Case 10-4: Labial Excision

OPERATIVE REPORT

LOCATION: Inpatient, Hospital

PATIENT: Mary Brown

ATTENDING PHYSICIAN: Andy Martinez, MD

SURGEON: Andy Martinez, MD

PREOPERATIVE DIAGNOSIS: Vulvar intraepithelial neoplasia III of the right labia.

POSTOPERATIVE DIAGNOSIS: Vulvar intraepithelial neoplasia III of the right labia.

PROCEDURE PERFORMED: Radical excision, right labia.

PREAMBLE: The patient is a 47-year-old woman who presented with a right labial lesion. This was biopsied and reported as being VIN-III; invasion cannot be ruled out. The decision was therefore made to proceed with radical excision of the right vulva.

PROCEDURE: The patient was taken to the operating room and general anesthetic was administered. The patient was then prepped and draped in the usual manner in lithotomy position, and the bladder was emptied with a straight catheter. The vulva was then inspected. On the right labia majora at approximately the 11-o'clock position, there was a multifocal lesion present. A marking pen was then used to mark out an elliptical incision leaving a 1-cm border on all sides. The skin ellipse was then excised using the knife. Bleeders were cauterized with electrocautery. A running locked suture of 2–0 Vicryl was then placed in the deeper tissues. The skin was finally reapproximated with 4–0 Vicryl in an interrupted fashion. Good hemostasis was thereby achieved. The patient tolerated this procedure well. There were no complications. Estimated blood loss was 75 cc.

Pathology Report Later Indicated: Neoplasia III, carcinoma in situ.

CPT Code(s): ______________________________

ICD-10-CM Code(s): ______________________________

ICD-9-CM Code(s): ______________________________

Abstracting Questions

1. In what area of the female genital anatomy is the labia located? ______________________________
2. CPT code assignment was affected by the extent (partial/complete) and what other factor? ______________________________
3. Define "in situ." ______________________________

Case 10-5: Dilation and Curettage

LOCATION: Outpatient, Hospital

PATIENT: Jenny Price

ATTENDING PHYSICIAN: Andy Martinez, MD

SURGEON: Andy Martinez, MD

PREOPERATIVE DIAGNOSIS: Menorrhagia.

POSTOPERATIVE DIAGNOSES
1. Menorrhagia.
2. Endometrial polyps.

PROCEDURE PERFORMED: Dilatation and curettage of the uterus and hysteroscopy.

ANESTHESIA: General.

SURGICAL INDICATIONS: This patient is a 35-year-old female who has been having prolonged and heavy bleeding. Ultrasound had suggested thickened endometrium.

OPERATIVE FINDINGS: On pelvic exam under anesthesia, the uterus was anterior upper normal size and firm. Adnexa revealed no masses. The uterus was 8.5 cm deep on sounding. She had a few small endometrial polyps in the lower uterine segment. Both tubal ostia were easily visualized.

DESCRIPTION OF PROCEDURE: After induction of general anesthesia, the patient was placed in the dorsolithotomy position, after which the perineum and vagina were prepped, the bladder straight catheterized, and the patient draped. After bimanual examination was performed, a weighted speculum was placed in the vagina, and the anterior lip of the cervix was grasped with a single tooth tenaculum. An endocervical curettage was then done with a Kevorkian curet. The uterus was then sounded to 8.5 cm. The endocervical canal was dilated to 7 mm with Hegar dilators. At 5.5 mm, an Olympus hysteroscope was introduced using LR as the distension medium. The cavity was systematically inspected and the above findings noted. The hysteroscope was withdrawn and the cervix further dilated to 10 mm. Polyps forceps was introduced and a few small polyps were removed. These were sent separately. Sharp endometrial curettage was then done. The hysteroscope was then reinserted and the polyps had essentially been removed. Blood loss was 5-10 cc. Specimen to pathology: endocervical curettings, endometrial curettings, and endometrial polyps. The patient tolerated the procedure well and returned to the recovery room in stable condition.

Pathology Report Later Indicated: Endocervical curettings, benign; endometrial curettings, benign; and endometrial polyps, benign.

CPT Code(s): ________________________________

ICD-10-CM Code(s): ________________________________

ICD-9-CM Code(s): ________________________________

Abstracting Questions

Review Case 10-2

1. How does this case differ from Case 10-2? ______________________________

Case 10-6: Cervical Cerclage Preoperative Examination

LOCATION: Outpatient, Clinic

PATIENT: Chandelle Jackson

ATTENDING PHYSICIAN: Andy Martinez, MD

SURGEON: Andy Martinez, MD

ADMITTING DIAGNOSIS: Decreased cervical length with suspected incompetent cervix.

PROCEDURE PLANNED: Cervical cerclage.

HISTORY OF PRESENT ILLNESS: The patient is a 26-year-old woman, gravida 5, para 2, whose last menstrual period was August 12 of this year, giving her an estimated date of confinement of May 17 of next year. This presently places her at 19 weeks and 3 days gestation. Her due date has been confirmed by pelvic ultrasound, the earliest of which was at 15 weeks gestation. We suspect possible incompetent cervix. The patient does have a history of two preterm deliveries, the first was 3 years ago in March when she delivered at 32 weeks after a 7-hour labor. Her previous obstetrician had therefore discussed with her that perhaps a cervical cerclage would be appropriate. Her history did not seem overly convincing for incompetent cervix. She had had LEEP procedure about 5 years ago. She then had a miscarriage the following year, for which she had a D&C, and then had a therapeutic abortion 2 years later. I have been following cervical length on this pregnancy. On initial scan at 15 weeks' gestation, cervical length was not performed but a week later was found to be 2.7 cm. Follow-up ultrasound done at 17 weeks' gestation showed cervical length to be 3.1 cm. The most recent ultrasound from 19 weeks' gestation showed cervical length decreased to 2.5 cm, and with the patient's questionable history the decision has been made to proceed with cervical cerclage.

OBSTETRIC AND GYNECOLOGIC HISTORY: As noted above.

PAST MEDICAL AND SURGICAL HISTORY: The patient had a tonsillectomy at age 14 and a hallex vagus correction at age 20.

MEDICATIONS: Prenatal vitamins.

PHYSICAL EXAMINATION: Blood pressure: 108/60. Height: 5′6″. Weight: 132 lb. Lungs: Clear to auscultation bilaterally. Heart: Sounds normal. Abdomen: Gravid with uterus palpable at the level of the umbilicus. Fetal heart rate is in the 140s. Bimanual examination was carried out, and the cervix is long, soft, and closed.

ASSESSMENT AND PLAN: The patient has had two previous preterm deliveries with history questionable for incompetent cervix, and now has decreased cervical length of 2.5 cm on ultrasound at 19 weeks' gestation. After discussing risks and alternatives, the patient has consented to proceed with cervical cerclage. She is aware of the risks, such as general anesthetic, hemorrhage, infection, ruptured membranes, and ultimately loss of the pregnancy. She does, however, consent to proceed, and the surgery has been scheduled for tomorrow.

CPT Code(s): ______________________________

ICD-10-CM Code(s): ______________________________

ICD-9-CM Code(s): ______________________________

Abstracting Questions

1. What section of the CPT would be referenced to locate a code to report the service provided in this report?

 ____

2. Was the patient admitted to the hospital after the clinic examination? ____________________

Case 10-7: Suction Dilation and Curettage

LOCATION: Inpatient, Hospital

PATIENT: Betsy Hall

ATTENDING PHYSICIAN: Andy Martinez, MD

SURGEON: Andy Martinez, MD

PREOPERATIVE DIAGNOSIS: Missed abortion with fetal demise, first trimester.

POSTOPERATIVE DIAGNOSIS: Same.

PROCEDURE PERFORMED: Suction D&C.

ANESTHESIA: General mask.

ESTIMATED BLOOD LOSS: 150 cc.

FLUIDS: 1000 cc.

COMPLICATIONS: None.

FINDINGS: Consistent with preoperative diagnosis.

PROCEDURE: The patient was prepped and draped in a lithotomy position under general mask anesthesia, and the bladder was straight catheterized, a weighted speculum placed in the vagina. The anterior lip of the cervix was grasped with single-tooth tenaculum. The uterus was then sounded to a depth of 8 cm. The cervical os was then serially dilated to allow passage of a size 10 curved suction curette, which was then used to evacuate intrauterine contents. A sharp curette was then used to gently palpate the uterine wall with negative return of tissue, and the suction curette was again used with negative return of tissue. The tenaculum was removed from the cervix. The tenaculum site was oversewn with 3–0 chromic interrupted suture. The speculum was removed from the vagina. All sponges and needles were accounted for at the completion of the procedure. The patient left the operating room in apparent good condition, having tolerated the procedure well.

CPT Code(s): ____________________

ICD-10-CM Code(s): ____________________

ICD-9-CM Code(s): ____________________

Abstracting Questions

1. What was the reason this procedure was performed? ____________________
2. What factor affects ICD-10-CM abortion code assignment? ____________________
3. What factor affects ICD-9-CM abortion code assignment? ____________________

Case 10-8: Cesarean with Tubal Ligation

Dr. Martinez will provide only the delivery service and tubal ligation. The patient's hometown physician provided the antepartum care and will also provide the postpartum care.

LOCATION: Inpatient, Hospital

PATIENT: Melissa Houtena

ATTENDING PHYSICIAN: Andy Martinez, MD

SURGEON: Andy Martinez, MD

PREOPERATIVE DIAGNOSES
1. Three prior cesarean section deliveries.
2. Voluntary sterilization.

POSTOPERATIVE DIAGNOSIS: Same as Preoperative.

PROCEDURES PERFORMED
1. Repeat lower segment transverse cesarean section.
2. Bilateral Pomeroy tubal ligation.

ANESTHESIA: General.

PREAMBLE: The patient is a 30-year-old woman, gravida 4, para 3, at 36 weeks and 2 days gestation who presented initially to her hometown obstetrician in spontaneous labor. Because of her previous cesarean sections, she was transferred here. She was scheduled to have a repeat cesarean section. She also has expressed a desire for permanent sterilization and has signed the papers for a tubal ligation. She was sure of her decision to proceed with the tubal ligation. When she presented she was contracting every 2 minutes with moderate intensity. The cervix was not yet dilating, but with the intensity of contractions a decision was made to proceed with cesarean section for delivery.

PROCEDURE NOTE: The patient was taken to the operating room and a spinal anesthetic was administered. The patient was then prepped and draped in the usual manner in supine position with left lateral tilt. A Foley catheter was placed.

A Pfannenstiel skin incision was made superior to the pre-existing scar. The fascia was then transversely incised. Peritoneal cavity was then carefully entered as the bladder was pulled up quite high anteriorly. The bladder was then taken away from the front of the uterus and reflected out of the way using the bladder retractor. A transverse incision was then made in the lower uterine segment, and there was delivery of a liveborn male infant with Apgar of 8 at 1 minute and 10 at 5 minutes and weight of 5 lb 8 oz. The baby was suctioned on the table and immediately handed to the neonatal intensive care team. The placenta was then manually removed and appeared to be intact. At this point the uterus was exteriorized to allow for better visualization. The uterine incision was closed in a single running locked layer of 0 Chromic. Good hemostasis was achieved.

At this point attention was directed toward the fallopian tube. Both ovaries and fallopian tubes were identified and appeared to be completely normal. Fallopian tubes were grasped using Babcock clamps, and bilateral Pomeroy tubal ligation was carried out by tying off a loop of tube with plain suture and then excising the intervening portion of fallopian tube bilaterally. Good hemostasis of the fallopian tubes was ensured.

At this point the uterus was replaced within the peritoneal cavity. Pericolonic gutters were swabbed free of blood and clots. The uterine incision was once again inspected and confirmed to be hemostatic. The fascia was then closed using running 0 Vicryl. Finally, skin was reapproximated using 4–0 Vicryl in a subcuticular manner.

The patient tolerated this procedure well and went to the recovery room in good condition. There were no complications. The estimated blood loss was 300 cc. The patient received Ancef 1 gram IV after cord clamping.

CPT Code(s): ______________________________

ICD-10-CM Code(s): ______________________________

ICD-9-CM Code(s): ______________________________

Abstracting Questions

1. Was the tubal ligation reported separately? ______________________________
2. Was the history of previous c-section reported? ______________________________
3. Would a Z code/V code be required for the tubal ligation? ______________________________

Case 10-9: Cesarean Section

Dr. Martinez will be providing the postpartum care for this patient.

LOCATION: Inpatient, Hospital

PATIENT: Glenda Freemont

ATTENDING PHYSICIAN: Andy Martinez, MD

SURGEON: Andy Martinez, MD

PREOPERATIVE DIAGNOSIS: Intrauterine pregnancy at 31 weeks and 2 days.

POSTOPERATIVE DIAGNOSIS: Same as Preoperative.

PROCEDURE PERFORMED: Primary low transverse cervical cesarean section.

ANESTHESIA: General endotracheal.

SURGICAL INDICATIONS: The patient is a 26-year-old gravida 3, para 2, at 31 weeks and 2 days by menstrual dates, who presents with uterine bleeding. She had an apparent abruption on ultrasound, and the vagina was filled with blood clot. For these reasons she was taken to surgery for an emergency cesarean section.

OPERATIVE FINDINGS: The infant is a female, born at 1006 hours, weighing 5 lb 1 ounce, with Apgar scores of 8 at 1 minute and 9 at 5 minutes. There was a lot of blood in the uterine cavity and some adherent clot to the placenta, estimated to be less than a 10% abruption. The tubes and ovaries were normal.

PROCEDURE: The abdomen was prepped and draped. A Foley catheter was in. The patient was then given a general endotracheal anesthetic and the abdomen was opened through a Pfannenstiel incision. The bladder flap was opened transversely with scissors, and the bladder was dissected downward bluntly with a hand. A small incision was made in the myometrium of the lower uterine segment, and then entry into the uterus was accomplished bluntly with a Kelly clamp. Low transverse incision was made with bandage scissors. The infant was delivered without undue difficulty. The infant's mouth and nose were suctioned with a bulb syringe, the cord was clamped and cut, and the infant was handed to the intensive neonatal team. A segment of cord was taken for cord blood gases, and the placenta was then delivered manually. Inspection of the uterine incision revealed there was a brisk bleeder near the left corner of the incision, and this was oversewn initially, with the first layer a running locked 0 Vicryl and the second layer a running horizontal Lembert 0 Vicryl. The pelvis was irrigated with saline. The uterine incision was inspected and there was small amount of oozing from the incision, which was controlled with a singular figure-of-eight 0 Vicryl. When hemostasis was adequate and lap sponges were correct, attention was directed toward closure. The peritoneum was loosely approximated in the midline with a couple of mattress sutures of 2–0 Vicryl. A medium Hemovac drain was placed subfascially to exit below the right side of the incision. The fascia was closed with running 0 Vicryl using two strands, one from either side to the middle and tied independently. The skin was closed with staples and the drain sutured to the skin with silk. Estimated blood loss was 1200-1500 cc.

Specimen to pathology was placenta. Final sponge and needle counts were correct.

Pathology Report Later Indicated: Normal placental tissue.

CPT Code(s): ______________________________

ICD-10-CM Code(s): ______________________________

ICD-9-CM Code(s): ______________________________

Abstracting Questions

1. What trimester is 31 weeks and 2 days? ______________________________
2. What does gravida 3, para 2 mean? ______________________________

Case 10-10: OB Ultrasound

LOCATION: Inpatient, Hospital

PATIENT: Melody Blithe

ATTENDING PHYSICIAN: Andy Martinez, MD

RADIOLOGIST: Morton Monson, MD

EXAMINATION: Limited OB ultrasound.

CLINICAL SYMPTOMS: Heavy bleeding; pain; third trimester, approximately 32 weeks.

LIMITED OB ULTRASOUND: This is a limited evaluation to evaluate the placenta. The placenta is noted to be anterior. There is a focal hypoechoic area seen along the inferior margin of the placenta. This measures approximately 1.6 × 1.2 × 1.5 cm. This is at the edge of the placenta, which appears to be separating from the uterine wall, consistent with an area of abruption. Fetal presentation is cephalic. No placenta previa is seen. Fetal cardiac activity is 148 beats per minute.

Dr. Martinez was present for the examination and was aware of the findings. The patient will be taken to the operating room immediately for cesarean section.

CPT Code(s): ______________________________

ICD-10-CM Code(s): ______________________________

ICD-9-CM Code(s): ______________________________

Abstracting Questions

1. What code range was reviewed in the CPT manual to report the ultrasound? ______________________________
2. What factor in this report determines the correct CPT ultrasound code? ______________________________
3. Why would the heavy bleeding not be reported? ______________________________

Case 10-11: Laparoscopic Drainage of Cyst

OPERATIVE REPORT

LOCATION: Inpatient, Hospital

PATIENT: Patti Bryan

ATTENDING PHYSICIAN: Ronald Green, MD

SURGEON: Andy Martinez, MD

PREOPERATIVE DIAGNOSIS: Large left ovarian cyst.

POSTOPERATIVE DIAGNOSIS: Large left ovarian cyst.

PROCEDURE PERFORMED: Laparoscopic drainage of left paratubal cyst.

PREAMBLE: The patient is a 27-year-old woman found to have a large left ovarian cyst on ultrasound. This cyst was measuring up to 8 cm, and there was thought to be at least one septation within it. The patient was having increasing problems with irregular menses along with increasing left lower quadrant pain. The decision was therefore made to proceed with laparoscopy with the aim of draining this ovarian cyst.

PROCEDURE: The patient was taken to the operating room and general anesthetic was administered. The patient was then prepped and draped in the usual manner in the lithotomy position, and bladder was drained with straight catheter.

Speculum was placed to allow for visualization of the cervix, which was grasped anteriorly using single-toothed tenaculum. Cohen cannula was then placed to allow for manipulation of the uterus. At this point, gloves were changed and attention was directed toward the abdomen. An umbilical incision was made to allow for insertion of the Veress needle. This was done without incident, and the abdomen was then insufflated with 3 liters of carbon dioxide. A 10-mm trocar was then placed through the umbilical incision without incident.

At this point the pelvis was inspected. Immediately apparent was a large, simple-appearing cyst occupying the majority of the pelvis. In fact, it was impossible to get around the cyst to be able to inspect or identify the remainder of the pelvic organs. At this point a 5-mm trocar was then placed suprapubically. At time of trocar incision, a small puncture was made in the cyst itself. Clear fluid began draining from the cyst cavity. An aspirator was then placed within the cyst cavity, and approximately 150 cc of absolutely clear fluid was drained from the cyst. Puncture site was not bleeding. Once the cyst was deflated, the rest of the pelvis could be inspected. The uterus appeared completely normal. Right ovarian and fallopian tubes were visualized and appeared completely normal. On the left side, the left ovary was completely normal. This cyst was found to arise in the paratubal region and was not ovarian in origin. The cyst was nicely deflated, and as it was paratubal, the cyst was not excised. It was confirmed to be hemostatic. Remaining fluid was then aspirated from the cul-de-sac. The cul-de-sac appeared completely normal. Upper abdomen was inspected and was normal. Appendix was visualized and was also normal. At this point the procedure was terminated. The suprapubic trocar was removed, and good hemostasis was ensured. Abdomen was desulfated, and umbilical trocar was removed. The incisions were then closed using 4–0 Vicryl in a subcuticular fashion. Vaginal instruments were then removed, and cervix was confirmed to be hemostatic.

The patient tolerated the procedure well. There were no complications. Estimated blood loss was minimal.

Pathology Report Later Indicated: No malignancy.

CPT Code(s): ______

ICD-10-CM Code(s): ______

ICD-9-CM Code(s): ______

Abstracting Questions

1. What approach was utilized for this procedure? ______
2. Was the cyst removed? ______

Chapter 11
Orthopedics

Case 11-1: Arthroplasty and Spur Excision

LOCATION: Outpatient, Hospital

PATIENT: Merry Hoffert

PRIMARY CARE PHYSICIAN: Frank Gaul, MD

SURGEON: Mohomad Almaz, MD

PREOPERATIVE DIAGNOSIS: Arthritis, secondary impingement, right ankle.

POSTOPERATIVE DIAGNOSES
1. Osteoarthritic change, grade 3/4 tibia, medial shoulder of the talus, right ankle.
2. Osteophytic spurring with secondary impingement, both hard and soft tissue anterior talotibial articulation, right ankle.
3. Impinging soft tissue entity, anterolateral aspect of the ankle.

PROCEDURES PERFORMED
1. Abrasion arthroplasty, right ankle.
2. Excision of osteoarthritic spurs of the anterior articular margin, distal tibia.

PROCEDURE: After a satisfactory level of general anesthesia and the patient in a supine position, the extremity was prepped and draped in a routine sterile manner. At this time we proceeded with the establishment of routine arthroscopic portals. We entered from an anteromedial direction with camera, anterolateral direction with camera, and anterolateral direction with in-cutting device. At this setting there was a proud prominence of secondary scar tissue formation. We proceeded with its resection at this time. There were also areas of secondary eburnation change diffusely of grade 2/3 about the lateral aspect of the talus and focally grade 3/4 changes about the medial shoulder of the talus and the tibia as they articulate. There was also the demonstration with dorsiflexion of secondary abutment of soft tissue and proud tibial spurring. At this setting, with use of mechanical in-cutting device, we reamed back the abutment of the diarticular tibia and also at this time proceeded with abrasion chondroplasty and arthroplasty procedures where appropriate of the distal articular tibial plafond and the talus proper.

Medial and lateral recesses were evaluated at this time and were otherwise unremarkable. The posterior confines of the ankle other than the areas of graded arthritic change as noted above were otherwise unremarkable. With completion of this element of the procedure we simply proceeded with closure of portal sites. Both preprocedure and postprocedure arthroscopic photos were obtained for documentation purposes. The patient tolerated the procedure well and was transported to the recovery room in a stable manner.

CPT Code(s): ____________________

ICD-10-CM Code(s): ____________________

ICD-9-CM Code(s): ____________________

Abstracting Questions

1. What approach was used for this procedure? ____________________
2. Was the procedure limited or extensive? ____________________

Case 11-2: Meniscectomy, Knee

LOCATION: Outpatient, Hospital

PATIENT: Herbert Hoveland

PRIMARY CARE PHYSICIAN: Ronald Green, MD

SURGEON: Mohomad Almaz, MD

PREOPERATIVE DIAGNOSIS: Internal derangement of left knee.

POSTOPERATIVE DIAGNOSIS: Discoid lateral meniscus with secondary tearing, left knee.

PROCEDURES PERFORMED: Partial lateral meniscectomy.

PROCEDURE: After a satisfactory level of general anesthesia, with patient in the supine position, the extremity was prepped and draped. At this time, routine arthroscopic portals about the left knee were established. The knee was obscured because of a prominent fat pad. There was some hemorrhagic nature to the fat pad and a plical entity that was also proud and redundant, and this time we simply proceeded with trimming these back for the sake of visualization. Patellar tracking was otherwise unremarkable. There was grade I arthritis change about the midcistern of the patella. The medial and lateral compartments of the knee had diffuse areas of grade I arthritis change. The medial meniscus at this time had a retained hematoma about the inframeniscal recesses but with no evidence of tearing of the meniscus or the meniscal synovial junction. Cruciate structures, anterior and posterior, were identified and otherwise unremarkable. There was a displaced bucket handle type of tear. Once this had been reduced about the lateral compartment proper, it was significant to note this was a discoid type of meniscus. Given this meniscal type of structure, the long oblique tearing of it and the chronic degenerative quality to it suggested preexisting mechanical disruption. We simply proceeded at this time with removal of the discoid meniscus tear. The margins of the lateral meniscus remaining were firm and stable. Lateral recess was otherwise unremarkable. At the completion of this element of this procedure we proceeded with therapeutic injection of a Marcaine preparation. The patient was transferred to the recovery room in a stable manner without compromising or complicating events.

CPT Code(s): ______________________________

ICD-10-CM Code(s): ______________________________

ICD-9-CM Code(s): ______________________________

Abstracting Questions

1. Does the specific meniscus (medial and/or lateral) affect CPT code assignment? ______________
2. Does the specific meniscus affect the ICD-10-CM/ICD-9-CM code assignment? ______________
3. What was the type of tear indicated in the report? ______________________________

Case 11-3: Plical Excision

LOCATION: Outpatient, Hospital

PATIENT: Sally Hedges

PRIMARY CARE PHYSICIAN: Alma Naraquist, MD

SURGEON: Mohomad Almaz, MD

PREOPERATIVE DIAGNOSIS: Traumatic injury, left knee, with loose body.

POSTOPERATIVE DIAGNOSES
1. Osteochondral defects, inferior medial aspect, left patella.
2. Cartilaginous loose body, left knee.

PROCEDURES PERFORMED: Diagnostic arthroscopy, plical excision and removal of cartilaginous loose body.

PROCEDURE: After satisfactory level of general anesthesia and the patient in the supine position, the extremity was prepped and draped. Routine arthroscopic portals about the left knee were established. On entering the confines of the knee, it was significant to note that there was 30 cc of frank sanguineous fluid, which was retained in a kidney basin, and there were multiple fat body globules demonstrated. At this setting, we proceeded with the irrigation of the knee to remove all retained hematoma from the patella proper at this time about the inferomedial border. The inferomedial border had an approximately 1 × 1-cm defect of the cartilaginous tissue, which was removed. This was at the true margin, and at this time its patella was visualized tracking. This did not cause abnormal mobility, either medially or laterally.

Fat pad was also excised at this time for the sake of visualization. There was also superior patellar plical entity, which was removed because of its looseness and redundancy. This did not destabilize the patella in any manner. Medial compartment at this time had some superficial grade 1 wear and tear changes. Meniscus was probed and palpated; otherwise the intra-articular notch was unremarkable. PCL and ACL were otherwise unremarkable. Lateral compartment had at this setting some superficially grade 1–type changes about the lateral tibial plateau. The meniscus was probed and palpated and was otherwise unremarkable.

Lateral recess at this time demonstrated cartilaginous loose body that was firmly adherent to the hematoma. At this time I simply removed the grasper. Otherwise, physical findings were unremarkable. At this setting, the portal site was closed and the area was injected with Marcaine preparation. The patient tolerated the surgery well and was transferred to the recovery room in a stable manner.

Pathology Report Later Indicated: Fat pad, unremarkable.

CPT Code(s): ______________________________

ICD-10-CM Code(s): ______________________________

ICD-9-CM Code(s): ______________________________

Abstracting Questions

1. Did you report the diagnostic arthroscopy? ______________________________
2. Should the hematoma within the joint be reported separately? ______________________

Case 11-4: Medial Meniscectomy, Knee

LOCATION: Outpatient, Hospital

PATIENT: Morrie Pearce

PRIMARY CARE PHYSICIAN: Leslie Alanda, MD

SURGEON: Mohomad Almaz, MD

PREOPERATIVE DIAGNOSIS: Internal derangement, right knee.

POSTOPERATIVE DIAGNOSIS: Right knee bucket handle medial meniscus tear.

PROCEDURES PERFORMED: Partial medial meniscectomy, right knee.

PROCEDURE: After a satisfactory level of general anesthesia and the patient in a supine position, the extremity was prepped and draped. Clinically, at this time routine arthroscopic portals were established. On entering the confines of the knee, there were plical and fat pad entities that obscured the view. These were removed for the sake of visualization. There were some grade 1/2 changes about the patella of arthritic quality. Furthermore, at this time in the medial compartment of the knee, there was a significantly large displaced bucket handle tear. The tear was reduced and at this time created mismatch about the inferior surfaces given the chronic degenerative quality of the meniscus. This required trimming back to a stable margin. There was also a radial element of tear from the outer circumference aspect inward leaving approximately a fourth of the remnant medial rim of the meniscus intact. Once the meniscus had been debrided to smooth margins for apposition, the mismatched width apposition, and the radial element of the tear, I believe that this was not satisfactory in facilitating healing with any higher degree of probability and at this time simply proceeded with its extraction, amputating both the anterior and the posterior elements of the meniscus, simply extracting this. The remnant of the rim was mechanically debrided. The interarticular notch was well visualized and otherwise unremarkable with probing and palpation of the meniscal structures.

Lateral compartment at this time had some superficial wearing about the lateral tibial plateau and the medial meniscus, but was otherwise unremarkable. The patient tolerated this procedure well and was transported to the recovery room in a stable manner once sterile dressings had been applied.

Pathology Report Later Indicated: Fat pad, unremarkable.

CPT Code(s): ____________________

ICD-10-CM Code(s): ____________________

ICD-9-CM Code(s): ____________________

Abstracting Questions

1. Describe the position of a patient in a supine position. ____________________
2. In this report, "grade 1/2 changes" refers to the extent of what changes? ____________________

Case 11-5: Steroid Injection

LOCATION: Outpatient, Clinic

PATIENT: Kim Ortega

PRIMARY CARE PHYSICIAN: Frank Gaul, MD

SURGEON: Mohomad Almaz, MD

PROCEDURE PERFORMED: Steroid injection.

INDICATIONS: Left shoulder subacromial bursitis.

PROCEDURE: This procedure was done in the procedure area in the hospital.

After obtaining consent, area of the left shoulder was prepped in the usual fashion with Betadine; 6 cc of 1% lidocaine with 1 cc of Kenalog was injected in the left subacromial bursa without difficulty. The patient tolerated the procedure well without immediate complications. There was moderate relief of pain afterward.

The patient was advised to call me if she experiences any signs of infection, such as fever, chills, erythema, or swelling. She will call me in 3 days and tell me how she is doing.

CPT Code(s): 20610

ICD-10-CM Code(s): ____________________

ICD-9-CM Code(s): ____________________

Abstracting Questions

1. What is the medical term for inserting a needle into a joint? ____________________
2. Would the joint into which the needle is inserted affect CPT code assignment? ____________________

Case 11-6: Open Reduction Internal Fixation

Assign an E code to indicate how this injury occurred in addition to the diagnosis and service codes.

LOCATION: Outpatient, Hospital

PATIENT: Gordon Matlock

PRIMARY CARE PHYSICIAN: Ronald Green, MD

SURGEON: Mohomad Almaz, MD

PREOPERATIVE DIAGNOSIS: Displaced interarticular fracture, left thumb metacarpal head.

POSTOPERATIVE DIAGNOSIS: Same as Preoperative.

PROCEDURES PERFORMED: Open reduction internal fixation, left thumb metacarpal head fracture, with insertion of two modular hand-set titanium screws.

ANESTHESIA: General.

PROCEDURE: The patient was brought to the operating room and a general anesthetic was induced. The left upper extremity was then prepped with Betadine and draped in a sterile fashion. He had 1 gram of Ancef preoperatively. The limb was exsanguinated and the tourniquet inflated to 250 mm Hg for 40 minutes. With 4× magnification loupes, we made a Chevron incision on the ulnar aspect of the MP joint. Dissection was carried down to the joint capsule from the extensor tendon, exposing the ulnar ward joint capsule. We then made an arthrotomy incision dorsally. We then found the bone fragment that did represent the dorsal ulnar aspect of the metacarpal head. It was out in the soft tissues. It had the ulnar collateral ligament attached to it. We then removed granulation tissue from both bone surfaces and relocated this fragment. We then provisionally pinned this with a 0.028 Kirschner wire. We thought that screw fixation would be the most adequate, and we used the 1.3-mm titanium screws from the modular hand set. We placed one from ulnar to radial and a second screw from more dorsal ulnar to dorsal radial. This produced excellent fixation of the fragment. The K-wire was removed. We then used the mini C-arm to confirm excellent position of the internal fixation and anatomic reduction of the fracture. We irrigated the wound with sterile saline and closed the joint capsule with interrupted 4–0 Vicryl suture, the extensor mechanism with 4–0 Vicryl suture, and the skin with interrupted 5–0 nylon suture. Next, a thumb spica compression hand bandage was applied with plaster splints.

The patient tolerated the procedure well. He went to the recovery room in excellent condition. He will be dismissed as an outpatient today with plans for follow-up back in the office in about 2 weeks.

CPT Code(s): 26746 ______________________

ICD-10-CM Code(s): ______________________

ICD-9-CM Code(s): ______________________

Abstracting Questions

1. What approach was utilized for the repair? ______________________________

2. Within this report, this indicates internal fixation was applied. ______________________________

3. Was a modifier appended to the CPT code assigned to this service? ______________________________

Case 11-7: Fascial Sling Arthroplasty

LOCATION: Outpatient, Hospital

PATIENT: Becky Wellington

PRIMARY CARE PHYSICIAN: Ronald Green, MD

SURGEON: Mohomad Almaz, MD

PREOPERATIVE DIAGNOSIS: Degenerative arthritis carpometacarpal joint, left thumb.

POSTOPERATIVE DIAGNOSIS: Same as Preoperative.

PROCEDURES PERFORMED: Fascial sling arthroplasty, left thumb.

ANESTHESIA: General.

PROCEDURE: The patient was brought to the operating room and a general anesthetic was induced. The left upper extremity was prepped with Betadine and draped in a sterile fashion. The limb was exsanguinated and tourniquet inflated to 250 mm Hg for 40 minutes. With 4× magnification loupes, we made a Chevron incision at the base of the thumb metacarpal. Dissection was carried down to the CMC joints, preserving subcutaneous nerves and vessels. We made a longitudinal arthrotomy incision and exposed the trapezium. We then morselized the trapezium and slowly removed the pieces with the rongeur. We carefully removed the entire trapezium, preserving the underlying FCR tendon. There was eburnated bone at the base of the first metacarpal. We then placed a drill hole through the base of the first metacarpal from its dorsal surface to its volar ulnar base. We opened this up to accept the tendon transfer. We next harvested the flexor carpi radialis tendon through two incisions, a short 1-cm incision over the tendon at the distal wrist flexor crease and an incision parallel to this 10 cm up the forearm at the myotendinous junction, where the FCR was transected at the floor of the thumb. Both volar forearm wounds were then closed with 5–0 nylon suture.

We next transferred the FCR tendon through the hole at the base of the first metacarpal, which effectively slung the first metacarpal up to the second metacarpal. We then pinned this to the second metacarpal with a 0.045 Kirchner wire bent and cut off outside the skin. We next sutured the tendon to the hole in the first metacarpal with 4–0 Vicryl sutures and packed bone graft into the hole to secure this. We then placed a 4–0 Vicryl suture in the floor of the wound, placed two Bunnell needles over the limbs of this, and then threaded the tendon onto this in an accordion fashion. We tied this Vicryl, pulled the tendon down into the defect, where the trapezium was excised, and filled this nicely. We then proceeded with capsular closure, imbrication of the capsule, and closed this with 4–0 Vicryl sutures. The appearance was excellent. We irrigated the wound with sterile saline and closed the skin with interrupted 5–0 nylon sutures. Next, we applied Xeroform, and a thumb spica compression hand bandage was then applied with plaster splints immobilizing the thumb. The tourniquet was released, and good circulation returned to the hand.

The patient tolerated the procedure well and went to the recovery room in excellent condition. She will be dismissed as an outpatient today with plans for follow-up back in the office in approximately 2 weeks.

DISCHARGE MEDICATION: Lorcet, 30 tablets.

Pathology Report: No specimen was sent.

CPT Code(s): ____________________

ICD-10-CM Code(s): ____________________

ICD-9-CM Code(s): ____________________

Abstracting Questions

1. On what area of the body was the arthroplasty performed? ____________________
2. Was the tendon transfer bundled into the arthroplasty? ____________________
3. Are modifiers reported with these procedures? ____________________

Case 11-8: Excision Bone Tumor

LOCATION: Outpatient, Hospital

PATIENT: Tyron Banks

PRIMARY CARE PHYSICIAN: Leslie Alanda, MD

SURGEON: Mohomad Almaz, MD

PREOPERATIVE DIAGNOSIS: Bone tumor, distal lateral right femur.

POSTOPERATIVE DIAGNOSIS: Same as Preoperative.

PROCEDURES PERFORMED: Excision bone tumor, distal right femur.

ANESTHESIA: General.

PROCEDURE: The patient was brought to the operating room and a general anesthetic was induced. Right lower extremity was prepped with Betadine and draped in a sterile fashion. The limb was exsanguinated, and tourniquet was inflated to 300 mm Hg for 25 minutes. Ioban drape was applied. A standard 4-inch longitudinal anterolateral incision was made beginning at the lateral patellar region and extending proximally. Dissection was carried down through the lateral parapatellar region and lateral parapatellar arthrotomy was performed. We entered down to the lateral femur where the tumor was palpable. This appeared to represent a chondroma on the lateral femur. We elevated the soft tissue and periosteum off of this and then used osteotomes to sharply excise this and gradually take this down to its base. It appeared to be bleeding normal bone, and at that point we did put bone wax on the bone. We then closed the periosteum with a running 0 Vicryl suture, then closed the fascia and joint with a running 0 Vicryl suture, and then closed the skin with a subcuticular 2–0 Vicryl suture and a running 4–0 Monocryl suture. Steri-Strips were applied with gauze dressing, Kling, ABD, Kerlix, and a Coban. The tourniquet was released, and good circulation returned to the leg.

The patient tolerated the procedure well. He will be dismissed as an outpatient today with plans for follow-up in the office in approximately 2 weeks.

DISCHARGE MEDICATIONS: Tylenol #3, 30 tablets.

Pathology Report Later Indicated: Benign neoplasm.

CPT Code(s): ______________________________

ICD-10-CM Code(s): ______________________________

ICD-9-CM Code(s): ______________________________

Abstracting Questions

1. From what body part was the bone tumor excised? ______________________________
2. Was a graft required to repair the defect? ______________________________
3. Was any fixation required? ______________________________
4. What report is required to correctly assign a diagnosis to the excision? ______________________________

Case 11-9: Carpal Tunnel Release

LOCATION: Outpatient, Hospital

PATIENT: Judy Trumpet

PRIMARY CARE PHYSICIAN: Frank Gaul, MD

SURGEON: Mohomad Almaz, MD

PREOPERATIVE DIAGNOSIS: Left carpal tunnel syndrome.

POSTOPERATIVE DIAGNOSIS: Same as Preoperative.

PROCEDURES PERFORMED: Endoscopic left carpal tunnel release.

ANESTHESIA: Local with IV sedation.

PROCEDURE: The patient was brought to the operating room and the left upper extremity was prepped with Betadine and draped in a sterile fashion. IV sedation was then induced. We marked out both portals proximally and distally, and injected each with 2 cc of 0.5% Marcaine. We incised the proximal portal, and bleeding points were cauterized. With 4× magnification loupes, we dissected down to the antebrachial fascia transversely, and a curved dissector was inserted into the carpal tunnel. The transverse carpal ligament was probed and cleared of synovium. We then entered the trocar and sleeve, hyperextended the arm over the wrist holder, incised the portal, and advanced the trocar and sleeve out the distal portal. We then removed the trocar and entered the endoscope. We had excellent visualization of the transverse carpal ligament throughout. We cleared any remaining synovium with the probe. Then we cut the distal 50% of the ligament with the knives and reversed the endoscope from distally to proximally and cut the proximal 50% of the ligament. We released any remaining antebrachial fascial bands with the triangular knife. We saw the transverse carpal ligament bowstring apart, confirming full release. We therefore removed the trocar and sleeve, split the antebrachial fascia proximally from the proximal portal, and closed each portal site with interrupted 5–0 nylon sutures. Xeroform and gauze dressing were applied with a light Kling dressing. The patient tolerated the procedure well.

The patient will be dismissed as an outpatient today with plans for follow-up at the clinic in approximately 7-10 days.

DISCHARGE MEDICATIONS: Darvocet-N 100, 20 tablets.

CPT Code(s): ______________________________

ICD-10-CM Code(s): ______________________________

ICD-9-CM Code(s): ______________________________

Abstracting Questions

1. What was the approach for this procedure? ______________________________

Case 11-10: Debridement of Chondromalacia

LOCATION: Outpatient, Hospital

PATIENT: Beth Mahoney

PRIMARY CARE PHYSICIAN: Ronald Green, MD

SURGEON: Mohomad Almaz, MD

PREOPERATIVE DIAGNOSES
1. Chondromalacia, left knee.
2. Torn left medial meniscus per MRI scan.

POSTOPERATIVE DIAGNOSIS: Chondromalacia, left knee.

PROCEDURES PERFORMED
1. Examination, left knee, under anesthesia.
2. Arthroscopy, left knee, with debridement of chondromalacia.

ANESTHESIA: General with endotracheal intubation.

FINDINGS: The patient was found to have significant chondromalacia in all three compartments. She had some bare bone on the femoral trochlear and significant fraying of the articular cartilage on the patella, as well as on the medial femoral condyle. The articular cartilage on the lateral femoral condyle was just frayed slightly, but no large flaps of articular cartilage were raised. She did, however, have some flaps of articular cartilage raised on the floor of the lateral compartment. I could not find any specific meniscal tears, but both medial and lateral menisci had fringe tags, which we removed.

The anterior cruciate ligament was intact.

PROCEDURE: Under general anesthesia the patient's left knee was examined. She had no effusion. The collateral ligaments were intact. Lachman test was negative, as was the pivot shift. McMurray test was negative. We then prepped the patient's left leg with Betadine and draped it in a sterile fashion. An Esmarch bandage was used to exsanguinate the leg, and a tourniquet on the thigh was inflated to 300 mm Hg. The total tourniquet time was about 35 minutes.

Three portals were used for this procedure. The first was placed along the superior anterolateral aspect of the knee, the second was placed along the inferior anterolateral aspect, and the third along the inferior anteromedial aspect of the knee. We distended the knee with lactated Ringer's solution. We examined the suprapatellar pouch and the medial and lateral gutters. We immediately noted significant chondromalacia involving the patellofemoral joint. There were large flaps of articular cartilage hanging off the articular surface of the patella and actually an area of bare bone on the trochlea, which was close to the lateral femoral condyle. We used the shaver to trim the articular cartilage, which was hanging from the subchondral bone. We trimmed the leading edge of the fat pad slightly as well.

I then examined the medial compartment and probed the medial meniscus. We could not identify a specific tear of the medial meniscus, although there were multiple fringe tags, which were removed with the shaver. She does have, however, significant chondromalacia involving the weight-bearing surface of the medial femoral condyle. There were flaps of articular cartilage that were loose and just laying on the subchondral surface. We used the shaver to trim these loose bits of articular cartilage.

We then examined the notch area and probed the anterior cruciate ligament. It was intact. We then examined the lateral compartment and probed the lateral meniscus. The lateral meniscus was intact, although there were several fringe tags, which were removed. She did have some raised flaps of articular cartilage on the lateral tibial plateau, and these were trimmed with the shaver. The articular cartilage in the lateral femoral condyle appeared to be in relatively good condition with only minor fraying.

At this point, we thoroughly irrigated the knee and looked for any remaining loose fragments. We then drained the knee and injected 80 mg of Depo-Medrol with 2 cc of 1% Xylocaine. The hardware was removed and the skin incisions were closed using 4–0 nylon suture. Sterile dressings were applied under a 6-inch Ace wrap.

She was then awakened and taken from the operating room in good condition, breathing spontaneously.

FINAL SPONGE AND NEEDLE COUNT: Correct.

MEDICATIONS: She was given IV Kefzol preoperatively, and she will be continued on Keflex for 5 days postoperatively as well. She will also be started on some aspirin postoperatively.

Pathology Report Later Indicated: Chondromalacia.

CPT Code(s): ____________________

ICD-10-CM Code(s): ____________________

ICD-9-CM Code(s): ____________________

Abstracting Questions

1. Was this a diagnostic or surgical arthroscopy? ____________________
2. What is chondromalacia? ____________________
3. Debridement of the chondromalacia is also referred to as ____________________.
4. Was the diagnosis for the meniscal tear reported? ____________________

Case 11-11: Excision of Mass, Bursa

LOCATION: Outpatient, Hospital

PATIENT: Brittany Lionel

PRIMARY CARE PHYSICIAN: Ronald Green, MD

SURGEON: Mohomad Almaz, MD

PREOPERATIVE DIAGNOSIS: Mass, left prepatellar bursa.

POSTOPERATIVE DIAGNOSIS: Same as Preoperative.

PROCEDURES PERFORMED: Excision of mass, left prepatellar bursa.

ANESTHESIA: Local infiltration with 1% Xylocaine, supplemented with IV sedation.

PROCEDURE: The patient was placed in the supine position on the operating room table. She pointed out the mass on the anterior aspect of her left knee, which was a very small mass, perhaps 2 or 3 mm in diameter. This bothers her when she kneels on her left knee, and she wanted it removed. We therefore marked it with a marking pen since it was not a large mass but was still nevertheless fairly easily palpable.

We then prepped her left knee with Betadine and draped it in a sterile fashion. She was given IV sedation. We then infiltrated the area around the mass with 1% Xylocaine. Once adequate anesthesia had been achieved, we exsanguinated the left leg with Esmarch bandage and inflated a tourniquet to 225 mm Hg. The total tourniquet time was about 6 minutes.

We created an incision in a longitudinal fashion directly over this mass and carried it down through the subcutaneous tissue. We very quickly found this mass, which was perhaps half the size of a pea (0.5 cm). It was fairly firm, and we sent it to pathology. It appears to be part of the left prepatellar bursa. We then excised some of the adjacent bursal tissue. We found this was located directly over the left patella and the patella was very visible underneath this mass. We then probed the area, looking for any other masses. We then thoroughly irrigated the area and closed the subcutaneous tissue with 2–0 Vicryl and the skin with 3–0 nylon suture. Pressure was applied to this area, and the tourniquet was released after 6 minutes of tourniquet time. We then applied a 4 × 4 dressing and an Ace wrap over this. She was then awakened and taken from the operating room in good condition, breathing spontaneously. The final sponge and needle counts were correct. She tolerated this procedure very well.

Pathology Report Later Indicated: Benign mass of left prepatellar bursa.

CPT Code(s): ________________________________

ICD-10-CM Code(s): ________________________________

ICD-9-CM Code(s): ________________________________

Abstracting Questions

1. What was the body location of the tumor? ________________________________
2. What was the size of the mass? ________________________________

Case 11-12: Excision of Mass, Finger

LOCATION: Outpatient, Hospital

PATIENT: Monica Slavianski

PRIMARY CARE PHYSICIAN: Alma Naraquist, MD

SURGEON: Mohomad Almaz, MD

PREOPERATIVE DIAGNOSIS: Mass, right long finger.

POSTOPERATIVE DIAGNOSIS: Mass, right long finger.

PROCEDURES PERFORMED: Excision of mass, right long finger.

ANESTHESIA: IV regional block supplemented with local infiltration of 1% Xylocaine.

FINDINGS: The patient was found to have a mass on the palmar aspect of her hand at the base of the long finger. This was actually almost at the metacarpophalangeal flexion crease or just proximal to this. This mass was sitting directly on the flexor tendon sheath and appeared to be consistent with a ganglion.

PROCEDURE: The patient had an IV regional block performed on her right hand and forearm, and a tourniquet was inflated on her right arm. We then prepped her right hand and forearm with Betadine and draped them in a sterile fashion. We found that the anesthetic was not quite adequate and supplemented the anesthesia with some local infiltration of 1% Xylocaine. We then created an incision in an oblique fashion just proximal to the metacarpophalangeal flexion crease of the base of the long finger on the palmar surface of the hand. We very carefully spread the soft tissue under the skin and came directly down to the flexor tendon sheath of the long finger. We noticed a mass sitting on the flexor tendon sheath, perhaps 2 or 3 mm in diameter. This appeared to be consistent with a ganglion. We elected to essentially excise the flexor tendon sheath on which the mass sat. We removed the mass and sent it to pathology. We then elected to incise the flexor tendon sheath much like a trigger finger release. The patient was able to flex and extend her fingers, and there was no catching at all.

We then thoroughly irrigated this area with saline and closed the skin using 4–0 nylon suture. A Xeroform dressing was applied under a bulky hand dressing with an Ace wrap. She was then taken from the operating room after the tourniquet was released after about 22 minutes of tourniquet time. She tolerated this procedure very well.

Pathology Report Later Indicated: Ganglion cyst.

CPT Code(s): ____________________

ICD-10-CM Code(s): ____________________

ICD-9-CM Code(s): ____________________

Abstracting Questions

1. Was the incision of the flexor tendon reported separately? ____________________

Case 11-13: Arthroplasty, Hip

LOCATION: Inpatient, Hospital

PATIENT: Lillian Thompson

PRIMARY CARE PHYSICIAN: Ronald Green, MD

SURGEON: Mohomad Almaz, MD

PREOPERATIVE DIAGNOSIS: Osteoarthritis, right hip.

POSTOPERATIVE DIAGNOSIS: Osteoarthritis, right hip.

PROCEDURE PERFORMED: Right porous-coated total hip arthroplasty using secure fit 54 cup and secure fit size 8 stem plus 28+0 neck length ball.

ANESTHESIA: General.

PROCEDURE: After suitable general anesthesia had been achieved, the patient was positioned with the left side down on the operating room table. The patient's right hip, thigh, and leg were then prepped and draped in the usual manner. Standard lateral approach was made. Anterior muscle flap was elevated off the trochanter, taking the anterior third of the gluteus medius, a portion of the gluteus minimus, and a very small portion of the anterior aspect of the vastus lateralis. Anterior capsulectomy was performed. Posterior capsulotomy was performed after the neck had been osteotomized and the head removed. Retractors were placed for acetabular exposure. The patient was noted to have superior osteophyte. This was partially resected. The acetabulum was then reamed sequentially from 46 mm to 54 mm. A 54-mm trial fit very well. A 54-mm secure fit cup was then pressfit into place, and excellent pressfit was achieved. No screws were used. The cross-fire polyethylene was then inserted with 10-degree overhang directly posteriorly and superiorly.

The canal was then prepared for the femoral stem. Good bone quality was noted. It was elected to go with porous-coated stem rather than cemented one. The tapered reamers were used to size 8. Rasping was used to size 8. Calcar rasp was then used. With the +0 neck length it looked like there was equal leg length, good stability, and good soft tissue tension. Rasp and trial head were then removed. Canal was irrigated. The actual size 8 secure fit stem was placed. A trial reduction was then performed with the +0 neck length. Again, good stability and good leg lengths were achieved. The actual 28-mm head was then applied, and the hip reduced. The wound was closed in layers after thorough irrigation. Two Hemovac drains were inserted. The skin was closed with staples. Dressing was then applied. The patient tolerated the procedure well and returned to the recovery room in stable condition.

Pathology Report Later Indicated: Bone morsels and chips, normal structure.

CPT Code(s): ______________________________

ICD-10-CM Code(s): ______________________________

ICD-9-CM Code(s): ______________________________

Abstracting Questions

1. What three factors were considered when assigning the CPT code for this procedure? ______________

Chapter 12

Otorhinolaryngology

Make sure to check evolve learning system for the latest content updates

Case 12-1: Tympanostomy

OPERATIVE PROCEDURE

LOCATION: Outpatient, Hospital

PATIENT: SueBeth Highland

ATTENDING PHYSICIAN: Gary Sanchez, MD

SURGEON: Gary Sanchez, MD

PREOPERATIVE DIAGNOSIS: Right Eustachian tube dysfunction; right chronic otitis media with effusion, plugged right tube.

POSTOPERATIVE DIAGNOSIS: Same as Preoperative.

OPERATIVE PROCEDURE: Right tympanostomy, tube removal, and replacement.

ANESTHESIA: General anesthetic by inhalational mask technique.

PROCEDURE: Following informed consent from the parents, the patient was taken to the operating room and placed supine on the operating table. The appropriate monitoring devices were placed on the patient, and general anesthesia was induced. The right ear was evaluated. The old tube was removed. It was plugged with wax. A myringotomy incision was made anterior to this. Mucoid effusion was then suctioned. The new tube was then placed. Topical antibiotic drops were applied.

The left ear was then evaluated. The tube was in good position and was patent; nothing further was done. The patient was then allowed to recover from general anesthesia and was transferred to the recovery room in good condition. She tolerated the procedure well.

CPT Code(s): ______________________________

ICD-10-CM Code(s): ______________________________

ICD-9-CM Code(s): ______________________________

Abstracting Questions

1. Is the removal of the old tube reported separately? ______________________
2. What factor affects code assignment for the tympanostomy? ______________________
3. Is the evaluation of the left ear reported separately? ______________________

Case 12-2: Direct Laryngoscopy

LOCATION: Outpatient, Hospital

PATIENT: Harold White

ATTENDING PHYSICIAN: Jeff King, MD

SURGEON: Jeff King, MD

PREOPERATIVE DIAGNOSES
1. Left true vocal cord mass.
2. Hoarseness.
3. Asthma.
4. Gastroesophageal reflux disease.

POSTOPERATIVE DIAGNOSIS: Same as Preoperative.

OPERATIVE PERFORMED: Direct laryngoscopy with use of operating microscope for excision of a left anterior true vocal cord mass.

ANESTHESIA: Endotracheal.

INDICATIONS: A 65-year-old male with chronic hoarseness. Examination reveals a mass involving the anterior portion of the left true vocal cord. The patient also has a history of asthma and reflux disease.

PROCEDURE: After consent was obtained, the patient was taken to the operating room and placed on the operating room table in the supine position. After an adequate level of general endotracheal anesthesia was obtained, the patient was positioned for direct laryngoscopy. The laryngoscope was placed in position. There were no lesions in the oropharynx or hypopharynx. This was placed into the suspension. The microscope was then brought in. An exophytic mass was noted involving the anterior third of the left true vocal cord extending to the area of the anterior commissure. Utilizing the forceps and the micro scissors, the mass was excised. Hemostasis was achieved with pledgets soaked with 1:100,000 units of epinephrine. The laryngoscope was then removed and the patient turned over to anesthesia. The patient tolerated the procedure well, and there was no break in technique. The patient was extubated and taken to the postanesthetic care unit in good condition.

Pathology Report Later Indicated: Adenocarcinoma, poorly diffused, primary.

FLUIDS ADMINISTERED: 1000 cc of RL

ESTIMATED BLOOD LOSS: Less than 5 cc.

PREOPERATIVE MEDICATIONS: 12 mg of Decadron and 20 mg of Pepcid IV.

CPT Code(s): ______________________________

ICD-10-CM Code(s): ______________________________

ICD-9-CM Code(s): ______________________________

Abstracting Questions

1. Was the laryngoscopy direct or indirect? ______
2. Does the use of the operating microscope affect code assignment? ______
3. What other factor affected code assignment? ______
4. The primary diagnosis was identified based on what report? ______
5. Do the diagnosis codes differentiate between true and false vocal cords? ______

Case 12-3: Myringotomy with Tympanostomy

LOCATION: Outpatient, Hospital

PATIENT: Daniel Briggstad

ATTENDING PHYSICIAN: Jeff King, MD

SURGEON: Jeff King, MD

PREOPERATIVE DIAGNOSES
1. Recurrent otitis media.
2. Retained right PE tube and granulation tissue.
3. Left otitis media with effusion.

POSTOPERATIVE DIAGNOSES
1. Recurrent otitis media.
2. Retained right PE tube and granulation tissue.
3. Left otitis media with effusion.
4. Right tympanic membrane perforation.

PROCEDURES PERFORMED
1. Removal of right PE tube and granulation tissue from the tympanic membrane.
2. Left myringotomy with tympanostomy tube placement.

ANESTHESIA: General inhalation.

SURGICAL INDICATIONS: A 4-year-old male with a history of bilateral PE tubes. Since extrusion of the PE tubes, he has had recurrent episodes of otitis media. There is also granulation tissue around the right PE tube.

PROCEDURE: After consent was obtained, the patient was taken to the operating room and placed on the operating table in supine position. After the adequate level of general inhalation anesthesia was obtained, the patient was draped in the appropriate manner for PE tube placement. Attention was first focused on the right ear. Utilizing an ear speculum and microscope, the external canal was cleared of cerumen. The retained extruded PE tube was removed from the tympanic membrane. In addition, granulation tissue was also removed. Subsequent examination shows a perforation of the posterior inferior area. There is no effusion. Due to the significant size of the perforation, no PE tube was placed. Attention was then focused on the left side. The ear canal was cleared of wet debris and cerumen. The tympanic membrane was noted to be opaque. The myringotomy incision was then placed in the anterior inferior quadrant. Serous effusion was suctioned. A bobbin tympanostomy tube was then placed without difficulty. Cortisporin otic suspension and a cotton ball were then placed.

The patient tolerated the procedure well, and there was no break in technique. The patient was awakened and taken to the postanesthesia area in good condition.

CPT Code(s): ______________________________

ICD-10-CM Code(s): ______________________________

ICD-9-CM Code(s): ______________________________

Abstracting Questions

1. Was the removal of the tube from the right ear reported? ______
2. Was the removal of the tube from the left ear reported? ______
3. What procedure was performed on the left ear? ______
4. What three modifiers were reported with the CPT codes assigned for this case? ______

Case 12-4: Adenoidectomy

OPERATIVE REPORT

LOCATION: Outpatient, Hospital

PATIENT: Julie Hague

ATTENDING PHYSICIAN: Gary Sanchez, MD

PREOPERATIVE DIAGNOSIS: Nasal obstruction, adenoid hypertrophy, bilateral inferior turbinate hypertrophy, left septal deviation.

POSTOPERATIVE DIAGNOSIS: Nasal obstruction, adenoid hypertrophy, bilateral inferior turbinate hypertrophy, left septal deviation.

PROCEDURE PERFORMED: Adenoidectomy, bilateral inferior turbinate reduction.

ANESTHESIA: General endotracheal.

PROCEDURE: Following informed consent from the patient's mother, the 6-year-old child was taken to the operating room and placed supine on the operating table. The appropriate monitoring devices were placed on the patient, and general anesthesia was induced. She was orally intubated without difficulty. She was draped in the usual fashion. A mouth gag was carefully placed in the oral cavity and opened. A catheter was placed through the right nostril and brought out through the mouth and snapped so as to retract the soft palate. The nasopharynx was evaluated with a mirror. It was seen to have a significant amount of hypertrophic adenoid tissue present. This was removed under direct vision with several sweeps of the adenoid curet. Sponges were then placed in the nasopharynx to allow for hemostasis.

The nose was then evaluated. It had pretty significant bilateral inferior turbinate hypertrophy. It also had a moderate left septal deviation. I did pack the nose with Afrin-soaked gauze. I removed it after 5 minutes. I used a butter knife to outfracture the inferior turbinates, and there was not a lot of movement laterally of the turbinates. I then used the needlepoint cautery to cauterize the anterior/inferior portion of the turbinates. Great care was taken on the left side not to accidentally cauterize the septal deviation. Following this, I did place a Doyle splint on the right side, and I used a Silastic sheet on the left side. Because of the left septal deviation I could not get a Doyle splint into the left side. The splint and Silastic sheet were sutured to the anterior left nasal septum.

The sponges were removed from the nasopharynx. There was still a small amount of bleeding going on, and thus it was necessary to use suction electrocautery on several points in the nasopharynx to allow for hemostasis. This was achieved.

Pathology Report Later Indicated: No malignancy.

CPT Code(s): ____________________

ICD-10-CM Code(s): ____________________

ICD-9-CM Code(s): ____________________

Abstracting Questions

1. Does the age of the patient affect the adenoidectomy code assignment? ________________
2. Was this a primary or secondary adenoidectomy? ________________
3. Were the tonsils also removed? ________________
4. What procedure was performed to correct the turbinate deformity? ________________
5. Does the number of turbinates fractured affect code assignment? ________________

Case 12-5: Tonsillectomy and Adenoidectomy

OPERATIVE REPORT

LOCATION: Outpatient, Hospital

PATIENT: Lois Rock

ATTENDING PHYSICIAN: Ronald Green, MD

SURGEON: Jeff King, MD

PREOPERATIVE DIAGNOSIS: Chronic tonsillitis, tonsil and adenoid hypertrophy, obstructive sleep apnea.

POSTOPERATIVE DIAGNOSIS: Chronic tonsillitis, tonsil and adenoid hypertrophy, obstructive sleep apnea.

PROCEDURE PERFORMED: Tonsillectomy and adenoidectomy.

ANESTHESIA: General endotracheal.

PROCEDURE: Following informed consent from the patient's parents, the 8-year-old patient was taken to the operating room and placed supine on the operating table. The appropriate monitoring devices were placed on the patient, and general anesthesia was induced. She was orally intubated without difficulty. She was draped in the usual sterile fashion. A mouth gag was placed in the oral cavity and opened. A catheter was placed through the right nostril and brought out through the mouth and snapped so as to retract the soft palate. The nasopharynx was seen to have a moderate amount of hypertrophic adenoid tissue present. This was removed under direct vision with several sweeps of the adenoid curet. Sponges were then placed in the nasopharynx.

The left tonsil was then grasped with a straight Allis and retracted medially. With the cautery set at 12 watts in the coagulation mode, it was dissected out from superior to inferior by creating a plane between the tonsil and its muscular bed. It was removed in one piece without any bleeding.

The right tonsil was then removed in an identical fashion to the left tonsil. There was no bleeding. The right and left tonsillar fossa were each then injected with approximately 3 cc of 0.5% Marcaine with 1:100,000 epinephrine. The sponges were then removed from the nasopharynx. Suction cautery was used to cauterize several points in the nasopharynx to allow for hemostasis, which was achieved.

The patient then had the mouth gag and catheter removed from the mouth and nose. Estimated blood loss was less than 5 cc. She was transferred to the recovery room in good condition.

Pathology Report Later Indicated: No malignancy, but chronic tonsillitis with hypertrophy of tonsils and adenoids.

CPT Code(s): ______________________________

ICD-10-CM Code(s): ______________________________

ICD-9-CM Code(s): ______________________________

Abstracting Questions

1. The Procedure section of the report indicated that the catheter was placed in the right nostril. Does this mandate the assignment of modifier -RT? ______________________________
2. Was the cautery of the bleeders reported separately? ______________________________

Case 12-6: Esophagoscopy with Dilation

LOCATION: Outpatient, Hospital

PATIENT: Mike Osborne

ATTENDING PHYSICIAN: Jeff King, MD

SURGEON: Jeff King, MD

PREOPERATIVE DIAGNOSIS: Dysphagia with inability to swallow.

POSTOPERATIVE DIAGNOSES
1. Dysphagia with inability to swallow.
2. Esophageal stricture.
3. Mild esophagitis.

PROCEDURE PERFORMED: Esophagoscopy with dilatation.

ANESTHESIA: General endotracheal.

SURGICAL INDICATIONS: This 63-year-old male was unable to swallow after eating lunch today. He had a similar episode a couple of years ago and then a couple of days ago; however, the inability to swallow resolved within couple hours. This time he has been unable to swallow for 6 hours, with regurgitation of water shortly after swallowing it.

PROCEDURE: After consent was obtained, the patient was taken to the operating room and placed on the operating room table in the supine position. After an adequate level of general endotracheal anesthesia was obtained, the patient was positioned for esophagoscopy. The esophagoscope was passed through the cricopharyngeus. Prior to that, examination of the pharynx, oropharynx, and hypopharynx did not reveal any abnormality. The esophagoscope was easily passed to approximately 38 mm, where a narrowed area was encountered. There was some superficial esophagitis seen. There was no foreign body seen or food impaction. As such, the esophagoscope was removed and dilation was then begun. This was done with the bougies up to a 60 French size and a 60-mm depth. After completion of this, an NG tube and oral gastric tube were placed to suction out the stomach. The esophagoscope was then repassed, and the scope easily passed now to 40 mm. The patient tolerated the procedure well, and there was no break in technique; the patient was extubated and taken to the postanesthesia care unit in good condition. Fluids administered were 800 cc of RL. Estimated blood loss was minimal. Preoperative medication: None.

CPT Code(s): ____________________

ICD-10-CM Code(s): ____________________

ICD-9-CM Code(s): ____________________

Abstracting Questions

1. What was the approach utilized in this procedure? ____________________
2. What diameter dilation was achieved? ____________________
3. Was a guidewire used? ____________________

Case 12-7: Cervical Node Excision

LOCATION: Outpatient, Hospital

PATIENT: Marvin Lotburg

ATTENDING PHYSICIAN: Jeff King, MD

SURGEON: Jeff King, MD

PREOPERATIVE DIAGNOSES
1. Superior mediastinal and cervical lymphadenopathy.
2. Left vocal cord paralysis.

POSTOPERATIVE DIAGNOSIS: Same as Preoperative.

PROCEDURE PERFORMED: Left neck deep cervical lymph node excisional biopsy.

ANESTHESIA: General endotracheal.

INDICATIONS: This is a 42-year-old male who developed hoarseness. Examination revealed a paralyzed left vocal cord. Subsequent CT examination of the chest and neck revealed significant adenopathy in the superior mediastinum as well as bilateral cervical lymphadenopathy, with the left worse than the right. The patient is now ready for cervical node biopsy for tissue diagnosis.

PROCEDURE: After consent was obtained, the patient was taken to the operating room and placed on the operating room table in the supine position. After an adequate level of general endotracheal anesthesia was obtained, the patient was positioned for surgery on the left neck. The patient was noted to have an enlarged left upper neck lymph node; the left neck was prepped with Betadine and draped in a sterile manner. A curvilinear incision was marked overlying the mass. The area was then infiltrated with 1% Xylocaine with 1:100,000 units of epinephrine. After several minutes, sharp dissection was carried down through skin and subcutaneous tissue. Superior and inferior subplatysmal flaps were elevated. The mass was noted to be underneath the sternocleidomastoid muscle. As such, the sternocleidomastoid muscle was mobilized away from it. The enlarged lymph node was then dissected away from surrounding tissue. Anteriorly this was dissected away from the carotid artery and posterior and inferior from the internal jugular vein. Hemostasis was achieved with bipolar cautery as well as silk ties. Subsequent frozen section indicated poorly differentiated carcinoma. The area was then irrigated with saline. There was no active bleeding. The wound was then closed in layers with the platysma and subcutaneous tissue approximated with interrupted 4–0 Vicryl suture. The skin was approximated with Dermabond. A dressing was then applied.

The patient tolerated the procedure well, there was no break in technique, and the patient was extubated and taken to the postanesthesia care unit in good condition. Fluids administered: 1600 cc RL. Estimated blood loss: Less than 20 cc. Preoperative medications: 1 gram Ancef and 12 mg Decadron IV.

Pathology Report Later Indicated: Left neck mass, excision indicated metastatic poorly differentiated adenocarcinoma.

CPT Code(s): ______________________________

ICD-10-CM Code(s): ______________________________

ICD-9-CM Code(s): ______________________________

Abstracting Questions

1. Was this an open procedure? ______________________________
2. Was the biopsy performed superficial or deep? ______________________________
3. Was the purpose of the procedure for excision only? ______________________________
4. How were the results of the biopsy known before the procedure was completed? ______________________________

Case 12-8: Septoplasty

Assign an external cause/E code to indicate how the injury occurred.

LOCATION: Outpatient, Hospital

PATIENT: Leann Heathchilds

ATTENDING PHYSICIAN: Jeff King, MD

SURGEON: Jeff King, MD

PREOPERATIVE DIAGNOSES
1. Nasal fracture.
2. Septal deviation.
3. Nasal obstruction.

POSTOPERATIVE DIAGNOSES
1. Nasal fracture.
2. Septal deviation.
3. Nasal obstruction.

PROCEDURES PERFORMED
1. Septoplasty.
2. Closed treatment of nasal bone fracture with stabilization.

ANESTHESIA: General endotracheal.

INDICATIONS: A 24-year-old female who sustained nasal trauma after being hit by a batted ball while playing softball. This resulted in a nasal bone fracture and significant septal deviation with associated nasal obstruction. The patient presents now for surgical treatment.

PROCEDURE: After consent was obtained, the patient was taken to the operating room and placed on the operating room table in the supine position. After an adequate level of general endotracheal anesthesia was obtained and the patient was draped in appropriate manner for nasal surgery, the patient's nose was packed with cotton pledgets soaked with 4% cocaine. After several minutes, 1% Xylocaine with 1:100,000 units of epinephrine was infiltrated into the septum bilaterally as well as into the nasal dorsum area. Nasal hairs were trimmed. Then using a right hemitransfixation incision, mucoperichondrium and mucoperiosteal flaps were elevated. The deviation portion of the cartilaginous bone was removed. After achieving hemostasis, the flaps were returned to normal position. Subsequent reinspection showed no residual deformity. Attention was then focused on the nasal bones. The right nasal bone was depressed, and the left nasal bone was deviated laterally. As such, using the Sayer elevator, the depressed nasal bone was pushed out, and then with lateral pressure on the left nasal bone, the nasal pyramid was brought to the midline. Subsequently, the hemitransfixation incision was closed with interrupted 4–0 chromic suture. A quilting suture of 4–0 plain gut was then performed. Silastic splints were then placed on both sides of the nasal septum and secured with nylon suture. The nose was then packed bilaterally. The packs consisted of a Merocel sponge covered with a gloved finger coated with Bacitracin ointment. This was infiltrated with local solution. An exterior nasal splint was then applied. Nasal dressing was applied.

The patient tolerated the procedure well, and there was no break in technique. The patient was extubated and taken to the postanesthesia care unit in good condition.

FLUIDS ADMINISTERED: 1500 cc of RL.

ESTIMATED BLOOD LOSS: Less than 25 cc.

PREOPERATIVE MEDICATIONS: 1 gram of Ancef and 8 mg of Decadron IV.

CPT Code(s): ______________________________

ICD-10-CM Code(s): ______________________________

ICD-9-CM Code(s): ______________________________

Abstracting Questions

1. Was the nasal fracture repair accomplished by means of open or closed manipulation? ____________
2. Was the fracture externally stabilized? ______________________________
3. What was the open procedure that was performed? ______________________________

Case 12-9: Mandibular Angle Fracture

Assign an external cause/E code to indicate how the injury occurred.

LOCATION: Outpatient, Hospital

PATIENT: Kevin Green

ATTENDING PHYSICIAN: Jeff King, MD

SURGEON: Jeff King, MD

PREOPERATIVE DIAGNOSIS: Left mandibular angle fracture.

POSTOPERATIVE DIAGNOSIS: Same.

PROCEDURE PERFORMED: Open treatment of left mandibular angle fracture with interdental fixation.

ANESTHESIA: General nasotracheal.

INDICATIONS: This is a 24-year-old male who was in an altercation and sustained trauma to his mandible. Examination and radiologic evaluation revealed a left mandibular angle fracture. The patient presents now for surgical treatment.

PROCEDURE: After consent was obtained, the patient was taken to the operating room and placed on the operating room table in supine position. After an adequate level of general anesthesia was obtained, the patient was positioned for treatment of the left mandibular angle fracture. Attention was first focused on the oral cavity. The oral cavity was irrigated. The patient was then placed into his normal occlusion and interdental fixation was applied. Two-millimeter screws were placed into the area just above the mandibular and maxillary incisors. Those areas were infiltrated with 1% Xylocaine with 1:100,000 units of epinephrine. An incision was made and then the bone exposed. Drill holes were made and the 2-mm screws placed. A 25-gauge wire was then utilized to place the patient into mandibular fixation with his normal occlusion. With the interdental fixation completed, the patient was then positioned for an external approach to the mandibular angle fracture. The patient was prepped with Betadine and draped in a sterile manner. A curvilinear incision was then outlined two fingerbreadths below the mandibular angle area. This area was then infiltrated with 1% Xylocaine with 1:100,000 units of epinephrine. Sharp dissection was then carried down through skin and subcutaneous tissues. Superior and inferior subplatysmal flaps were elevated. The marginal branch of the left facial nerve was identified and preserved. The mandibular angle was exposed by first cutting through the masseter muscle and then through the periosteum. The fracture site was exposed. The fragments were then brought into approximation. Two 4-hole 2-mm plates were then positioned, one superiorly and one along the border, and screwed in place. The area was then irrigated with antibiotic solution. The masseter muscle and periosteum were then reapproximated with interrupted 3–0 Vicryl suture. The wound was then closed in layers over a ¼-inch Penrose drain, with the platysma and subcutaneous tissue approximated with interrupted 4–0 Vicryl suture and the skin approximated with interrupted 5–0 nylon suture in a vertical mattress closure. Bacitracin ointment was applied. A dressing of Fluffs and Kerlix was then placed. The patient was then turned over to anesthesia.

The patient tolerated the procedure well, there was no break in technique, and the patient was extubated and taken to the postanesthesia care unit in good condition. Fluids administered: 2000 cc RL. Estimated blood loss: 75 cc. Preoperative medications: 900 mg Cleocin and 12 mg Decadron IV.

CPT Code(s): ______________________________

ICD-10-CM Code(s): ______________________________

ICD-9-CM Code(s): ______________________________

Abstracting Questions

1. Was treatment of the fracture open or closed? ______________________________
2. Was interdental fixation applied? ______________________________
3. Was the mandibular angle fracture an open or closed fracture? ______________________________

Case 12-10: Branchial Cleft Fistula Repair

LOCATION: Outpatient, Hospital

PATIENT: Lori Davison

ATTENDING PHYSICIAN: Jeff King, MD

SURGEON: Jeff King, MD

PREOPERATIVE DIAGNOSIS: Left branchial cleft fistula.

POSTOPERATIVE DIAGNOSIS: Same as Preoperative.

PROCEDURE PERFORMED: Excision of left branchial cleft fistula extending into the area of the left piriform sinus.

ANESTHESIA: General endotracheal.

INDICATIONS: This is a 20-year-old female who has had a draining pit in the left mid-neck, just anterior to the sternocleidomastoid muscle, since early childhood. The patient now desires definitive surgical treatment.

PROCEDURE: After consent was obtained, the patient was taken to operating room and placed on the operating table in the supine position. After an adequate level of general endotracheal anesthesia was obtained, the patient was positioned for surgery on the left neck. The patient's left neck was prepped with Betadine and draped in a sterile manner. The pit was noted in the junction between the superior ⅔ and inferior ⅓ of the neck just anterior to the sternocleidomastoid muscle. On compressing the upper portion of the neck, some drainage was noted from the pit. An ellipse of the skin was marked around the pit and then lateral extensions were made from there in the skin crease line. The area was then infiltrated with 1% Xylocaine with 1:100,000 units of epinephrine. Sharp dissection was carried down through the skin and subcutaneous tissue. A lacrimal probe was then carried down through the skin and subcutaneous tissue. This was dissected away from the sternocleidomastoid muscle as well as the strap muscles and the thyroid cartilage. Dissection was then carried superiorly. The dilator was removed and replaced with a Fogarty catheter. The balloon was inflated to identify the distal end. The fistula was then dissected to an area just behind the thyroid cartilage and the area of the piriform sinus. It did not extend into piriform sinus. As such, just distal to the end of the fistula tract, a clamp was placed, and then the specimen was removed. This was then ligated with 3–0 silk ties. Hemostasis was achieved with bipolar cautery. The area was then irrigated with saline. The wound was then closed in layers by reapproximating the platysma and subcutaneous tissue with interrupted 3–0 and 4–0 Vicryl suture. The skin was approximated with interrupted 5–0 rapid-absorbing gut suturing. Benzoin and Steri-Strips were applied. A pressure dressing of Fluffs and Kerlix was then placed.

The patient tolerated the procedure well. There was no break in technique. The patient was extubated and taken to the postanesthesia care unit in good condition.

FLUIDS ADMINISTERED: 1500 cc of RL.

ESTIMATED BLOOD LOSS: Less than 20 cc.

PREOPERATIVE MEDICATIONS: 1 gram of Ancef and 12 mg of Decadron IV.

Pathology Report Later Indicated: Soft tissue of left neck, excision: brachial cleft cyst.

CPT Code(s): ____________________

ICD-10-CM Code(s): ____________________

ICD-9-CM Code(s): ____________________

Abstracting Questions

1. Was the procedure performed only at the subcutaneous tissue level? ____________________
2. The Procedure Performed section of the report indicates the fistula extended into the area of the left piriform sinus. What is the piriform sinus? ____________________

Case 12-11: Incus and Stapes Mobilization

LOCATION: Outpatient, Hospital

PATIENT: Pat Zapata

ATTENDING PHYSICIAN: Jeff King, MD

SURGEON: Jeff King, MD

PREOPERATIVE DIAGNOSIS: Bilateral mixed hearing loss with significant conductive component in the lower frequencies, left ear worse than the right.

POSTOPERATIVE DIAGNOSES
1. Bilateral mixed hearing loss with significant conductive component in the lower frequencies, left ear worse than the right.
2. Left middle ear tympanosclerosis around the incus and stapes.

PROCEDURE PERFORMED
1. Left middle ear exploration.
2. Left incus and stapes mobilization.

ANESTHESIA: General endotracheal.

INDICATIONS: This is a 16-year-old female with a long history of hearing loss. Recent audiometric testing indicated bilateral mixed hearing loss with a significant conductive component in the lower frequencies. The left ear was worse than the right. The patient has used hearing aids but noted that the hearing aid is not as effective as it had been. As such, the patient's mother had opted for exploration to correct any ossicular abnormality if noted, with the exception of stapedectomy.

PROCEDURE: After consent was obtained, the patient was taken to the operating room and placed on the operating table in supine position. After an adequate level of general endotracheal anesthesia was obtained, the patient was positioned for surgery on the left ear. The patient's left ear was prepped with Betadine and draped in a sterile manner. One-percent Xylocaine with 1:100,000 units of epinephrine was infiltrated into the postauricular area and then in all four quadrants of the ear canal. The speculum was secured with a speculum holder. A tympanomeatal flap was then elevated in standard fashion. The ossicular chain was intact; however, the incus and stapes were not mobile. There was tympanosclerotic plaque around the incus and stapes. With meticulous dissection this was removed. Subsequently, the incus and stapes were mobile. The round window area showed that the niche was very deep, and the membrane could not be seen. Fluid was placed into the niche to see if a round window reflex could be elicited, but a clear obvious round window reflex was not elicited. The tympanomeatal flap was then placed back in its normal position. Gelfoam soaked with Physiosol was then placed lateral to this and brought out through the proximal ear canal. The proximal ear canal was then filled with Bacitracin ointment. A cotton ball coated with Bacitracin ointment was placed in the conchal bowl area and a Band-Aid dressing applied.

The patient tolerated the procedure well, there was no break in technique, and the patient was extubated and taken to the postanesthesia care unit in good condition. Fluids administered: 1000 cc RL. Estimated blood loss: Less than 5 cc.

CPT Code(s): ___

ICD-10-CM Code(s): ___

ICD-9-CM Code(s): ___

Abstracting Questions

1. Was the mobilization of the incus reported separately? ___
2. What procedure was the surgeon NOT authorized to perform? ___

Case 12-12: Ethmoidectomy, Sphenoidotomy, and Septoplasty

Ready for a challenge? This case will give your coding skills an excellent workout. There will be five service codes and five diagnosis codes. The most extensive procedure is the septoplasty, and that code will be sequenced first.

LOCATION: Outpatient, Hospital

PATIENT: Russell Price

ATTENDING PHYSICIAN: Jeff King, MD

SURGEON: Jeff King, MD

PREOPERATIVE DIAGNOSES
1. Septal deviation.
2. Bilateral sinonasal polyposis.
3. Pansinusitis.
4. Bilateral inferior turbinate hypertrophy.
5. Nasal obstruction.

POSTOPERATIVE DIAGNOSIS: Same as Preoperative.

PROCEDURES PERFORMED
1. Bilateral endoscopic total ethmoidectomy.
2. Bilateral endoscopic maxillary antrostomy with removal of polyps from maxillary sinus.
3. Bilateral endoscopic sphenoidotomy.
4. Septoplasty.
5. Bilateral inferior turbinate overfracture.

ANESTHESIA: Endotracheal.

INDICATIONS: A 43-year-old male with history of nasal trauma that resulted in a septal deviation. He also has a history of bilateral sinonasal polyposis and has undergone prior polypectomy and sinus surgery. The patient now has recurrent disease. This was confirmed on examination and the CT scan. He also has bilateral inferior turbinate hypertrophy. The patient also has a history of severe snoring. He is to undergo correction of his nasal obstruction and sinusitis to see if that will help. If not, further evaluation of his snoring will be done.

PROCEDURE: After consent was obtained, the patient was taken to the operating room and placed on the operating table in supine position. After an adequate level of general endotracheal anesthesia was obtained, the patient was positioned for nasal and sinus surgery. The patient's nose was packed with cotton pledgets soaked with 4% cocaine. After several minutes, 1% Xylocaine with 1:100,000 epinephrine was infiltrated into the nasal portion of the polyps as well as the septum bilaterally and the inferior turbinates. Nasal hairs were trimmed. Attention was first focused on the right side. Using the 5-degree sinuscope and the microdebrider, the nasal portions of the polyps were removed. Polyps were noted both medial and lateral to the middle turbinate. There was also some scarring from the middle turbinate to the lateral nasal wall. This scar tissue was also removed with a microdebrider. Subsequently, polyps in the middle meatus and anterior posterior ethmoid areas were removed with microdebrider.

The maxillary sinus ostia area was cleared of polyps, and then the ostium was widened in a posterior-to-inferior direction. Polyps within the sinus near the ostia were also removed. The area was then packed with cotton pledgets soaked with 1:50,000 units of epinephrine. Attention was then focused on the left side, where a similar procedure was performed. Again, polyps were noted to be both medial and lateral to the middle turbinate remnant. Polyps were obstructing the maxillary sinus drainage area and were also cleared. The left side was packed with a pledget soaked with epinephrine solution. Attention was refocused on the right side, where further polyps were removed from the sphenoid/ethmoid area. Remnant of the superior turbinate was also cleared of polyps. The sphenoid sinus ostium was cleared of polyps. The area was then packed with cotton pledget soaked with epinephrine solution. Similar procedure was then performed on the left side. Attention was then focused on the nasal septum. Utilizing a right hemitransfixion incision, mucoperichondrium and mucoperiosteal flaps were elevated. The cartilaginous septum was noted to be severely attenuated and deviated with several fractured areas. Deviated portions were removed. This does not leave much support for the nasal tip area. If this is a problem in the future, this will need to be reconstructed. The deviated portion of the bony septum and spurs off the maxillary crest were then removed.

Attention was then focused on the inferior turbinates, which were outfractured. The hemitransfixion incision was then closed with an interrupted 4–0 chromic suture. A quilting suture of 4–0 plain gut was then performed. The pledgets in the sinus area were then removed. There was some oozing from the ethmoid as well as the sphenoid sinus areas. As such, these areas were coated with FloSeal and then packed lightly with strips of Surgicel soaked with local solutions. Bacitracin ointment was then applied. Silastic splints were then placed on both sides of the nasal septum and secured with nylon suture. The nose was then packed bilaterally. Packs consisted of a Merocel sponge with a gloved finger coated with Bacitracin ointment. It was inflated with location solution. Nasal dressing was applied.

The patient tolerated the procedure well, and there was no break in technique. The patient was extubated and taken to the postanesthetic care unit in good condition. Fluids administered included 2000 cc RL. Blood loss was less than 150 cc. Preoperative medications included 12 mg Decadron and 1 gram Ancef IV.

CPT Code(s): ______________________________

ICD-10-CM Code(s): ______________________________

ICD-9-CM Code(s): ______________________________

Abstracting Questions

1. Maxillary Sinus
   a. Were polyps/tissue removed? ______________________________
   b. What additional work was done to this sinus? ______________________________
2. Sphenoid Sinus
   a. Were polyps/tissue removed? ______________________________
3. Ethmoid Sinus
   a. Were polyps/tissue removed? ______________________________
   b. Was this anterior, posterior, or both? ______________________________
4. Inferior Tubinates
   a. Was there specific work done on this area? ______________________________
5. What modifiers were appended extensively to the majority of CPT codes that reported the services provided in this case? ______________________________
6. What does the diagnosis "pansinusitis" indicate? ______________________________

Case 12-13: Tarsorrhaphy

OPERATIVE PROCEDURE

LOCATION: Inpatient, Hospital

PATIENT: Daniel Blue

ATTENDING PHYSICIAN: Gary Sanchez, MD

SURGEON: Gary Sanchez, MD

PREOPERATIVE DIAGNOSIS: Paralytic ectropion and corneal exposure, left eye.

POSTOPERATIVE DIAGNOSIS: Same as Preoperative.

PROCEDURE PERFORMED: Medial tarsorrhaphy, left eye.

ANESTHESIA: Local with intravenous sedation.

COMPLICATIONS: None.

ESTIMATED BLOOD LOSS: Minimal.

PROCEDURE: In the operating room, after intravenous sedation, the patient was given a total of about a 0.5 cc of local infiltrative anesthesia. The skin surfaces on the medial area of the lid medial to the punctum were denuded. A bolster had been prepared, and double-arm 5–0 silk suture was passed through the bolster, which was passed through the inferior skin and raw lid margin, then through the superior margin and out through the skin. A superior bolster was then applied. The puncta were probed with wire instrument and found not obstructed. The suture was then fully tied and trimmed. Bacitracin ointment was placed on the surface of the skin. The patient left the operating room in stable condition, without complications, having tolerated the procedure well.

CPT Code(s): ______________________________

ICD-10-CM Code(s): ______________________________

ICD-9-CM Code(s): ______________________________

Abstracting Questions

1. What was the term that will help you identify the correct CPT code for this tarsorraphy? ______________
2. What was the important term to report the correct diagnosis of ectropion? ______________

Chapter 13

Pathology

Make sure to check evolve learning system for the latest content updates

*Do **not** report the professional modifier -26 for the following reports.*

Case 13-1: L3-4 Disc

LOCATION: Outpatient, Hospital

PATIENT: Corrine Wilson

ATTENDING PHYSICIAN: Timothy Pleasant, MD

SURGEON: Timothy Pleasant, MD

PATHOLOGIST: Grey Lonewolf, MD

CLINICAL HISTORY: Lumbar disc L3-4 herniation.

SPECIMEN RECEIVED: L3-4 disc.

GROSS DESCRIPTION: The specimen is labeled with the patient's name and "lumbar disc L3-4" and consists of fibrillary pink-tan tissue fragments. Representative section in one cassette.

MICROSCOPIC DIAGNOSIS: Fragments of fibrocartilage, consistent with herniated disc L3-4.

CPT Code(s): ______________________________

ICD-10-CM Code(s): ______________________________

ICD-9-CM Code(s): ______________________________

Abstracting Questions

1. How would the code for this service be referenced in the CPT index? ______________________________
2. Was the examination gross, microscopic, or both? ______________________________
3. What was the level of surgical pathology? ______________________________
4. Does the pathologic status of the tissue affect the diagnosis code? ______________________________

Case 13-2: Uterus, Bilateral Tubes, and Ovaries

LOCATION: Outpatient, Hospital

PATIENT: Tina Highdorn

ATTENDING PHYSICIAN: Ira Avila, MD

SURGEON: Ira Avila, MD

PATHOLOGIST: Grey Lonewolf, MD

CLINICAL HISTORY: Menorrhagia.

SPECIMEN RECEIVED: Uterus, bilateral tubes, and ovaries.

GROSS DESCRIPTION: The specimen is labeled with the patient's name and "uterus, bilateral tubes, and ovaries" and consists of 370 gm; this includes the complete uterus with tubes and ovaries. The uterus measures 14 cm in length × 10 cm in fundal diameter. The specimen is distorted by several bulging areas on the surface. The cervix is transverse. The endometrium is up to 0.3 cm thick and composed of pale tan color. Cut section of the myometrium reveals multiple whirling masses, up to 3 cm in diameter, consisting of white whirling tissue. The fallopian tubes have been surgically divided. The left ovary measures 5 × 4 cm and contains a central cystic structure with smooth lining. A section of the left tube and ovary is placed in cassette labeled 7. The right ovary measures 3 × 2 × 1.5 cm and is composed of wrinkled tan tissue. A section of the right tube and ovary is placed in cassette labeled 8.

MICROSCOPIC DIAGNOSIS: Sections of cervix show squamous metaplasia. Sections of endometrium show tubular glands lined by pseudostratified columnar epithelium. Small nests of endometrial glands and stroma are noted in the superficial myometrium. Sections of myometrium show masses, consisting of interdigitating bands of smooth muscle. Section of left fallopian tube is unremarkable. Section of left ovary shows a follicle cyst. Sections of right fallopian tube are unremarkable. Section of right ovary shows physiologic structures.

DIAGNOSIS
Complete uterus, tubes, and ovaries showing:
1. Squamous metaplasia, cervix.
2. Proliferating endometrium.
3. Adenomyosis, uterus.
4. Multiple intramural leiomyomata.
5. Status post surgical division of fallopian tubes.
6. Follicle cyst, left ovary.

CPT Code(s): ______________________________

ICD-10-CM Code(s): ______________________________

ICD-9-CM Code(s): ______________________________

Abstracting Questions

1. When you reference "Metaplasia, cervix" in the Index of the ICD-10-CM you are referred to what code? In ICD-9-CM, the coder is directed to *"omit code."* What does this direction mean? ______________________
2. When "Metaplasia, cervix" is referenced in the Index of ICD-9-CM you are directed to "omit code." What does this mean? ______________________
3. The clinical history was menorrhagia. What is menorrhagia? ______________________
4. Why was it not correct to report menorrhagia as the diagnosis? ______________________

Case 13-3: Placenta

LOCATION: Inpatient, Hospital

PATIENT: Cindy Kretchenhoff

ATTENDING PHYSICIAN: Ira Avila, MD

SURGEON: Ira Avila, MD

PATHOLOGIST: Grey Lonewolf, MD

CLINICAL HISTORY: 31 weeks, 6 days' gestation, possible placental abruption.

SPECIMEN RECEIVED: Placenta.

GROSS DESCRIPTION: Submitted in formalin, labeled with the patient's name, and "placenta" is 600 gm. Discoid placenta measuring 18 × 17 × 3 cm, with three centrally attached vessels and 5 cm long umbilical cord. The umbilical cord shows no knots or gross abnormalities (cassette 1). The membranes are tan and opaque and show no significant exudates, nodules, or green discoloration (cassette 2). The fetal surface of placenta shows a normal vascular pattern. The maternal surface features multiple intact cotyledons. No significant adherent blood clot or cotyledon compression is seen. Sectioning reveals dark red to purple spongy parenchyma without significant scarlike areas or masses. Representative sections of central and peripheral placenta are submitted in cassettes 3 and 4, respectively (two separate specimens, placenta and umbilical cord).

MICROSCOPIC DIAGNOSIS: Sections are umbilical cord showing three vessels. No significant inflammatory infiltrates are seen. Sections of membranes feature intact chorionic and amnionic membranes. Focal mild neutrophilic infiltrates are identified within chorionic membranes. Sections of placenta show multiple chorionic villi with villous architecture consistent with 32 weeks' gestational age. Villous vascularity is within normal limits. There is mild intervillous fibrin deposition. No significant large vessels lesions are seen. Minimal neutrophilic infiltrates are present within the fibrin beneath the chorionic plate.

DIAGNOSIS: Placenta, delivery; early third-trimester placenta, membranes, and umbilical cord showing mild early placentitis.

COMMENTS: While no gross pathologic changes of placental abruption are seen, acute abruption may not be accompanied by demonstrable placental changes at the time of pathologic examination.

CPT Code(s): ______________________________

ICD-10-CM Code(s): ______________________________

ICD-9-CM Code(s): ______________________________

Abstracting Questions

1. How many specimens were examined? ____
2. According to the notes in the CPT manual before 88300, the unit of services for codes 88300 through 88309 is the what? ____
3. Also in the notes of the CPT manual before 88300, a specimen is defined as tissue(s) submitted for individual and separate attention, requiring individual examination and pathologic ______________________.

Case 13-4: Cervical Disc

LOCATION: Outpatient, Hospital

PATIENT: Sally Reagon

ATTENDING PHYSICIAN: Timothy Pleasant, MD

SURGEON: Timothy Pleasant, MD

PATHOLOGIST: Grey Lonewolf, MD

CLINICAL HISTORY: Severe cervical spinal stenosis.

SPECIMEN RECEIVED: Cervical disc.

GROSS DESCRIPTION: The specimen is labeled with the patient's name and "cervical disc" and consists of approximately 5 grams of tan fibrous fragments.

MICROSCOPIC DIAGNOSIS: Sections show disc tissue.

DIAGNOSIS: Disc tissue (cervical).

CPT Code(s): ________________________________

ICD-10-CM Code(s): ________________________________

ICD-9-CM Code(s): ________________________________

Abstracting Questions

1. What statement in the code description for 88304 identifies cervical disc pathological examination?

   ____

Case 13-5: Cervical Disc

LOCATION: Outpatient, Hospital

PATIENT: Mary Ann Severson

ATTENDING PHYSICIAN: Timothy Pleasant, MD

SURGEON: Timothy Pleasant, MD

PATHOLOGIST: Grey Lonewolf, MD

CLINICAL HISTORY: Cervical C5-6 disc herniation.

SPECIMEN RECEIVED: C5-6 disc.

GROSS DESCRIPTION: Submitted in formalin and labeled with the patient's name and "C5-6 disc" are fragments of ragged tan tissue measuring approximately 5 × 2 × 1 cm in aggregate. Representative fragments in one cassette.

MICROSCOPIC DIAGNOSIS: Intervertebral disc, C5-6, discectomy; fibrocartilaginous intervertebral disc, fragments of.

CPT Code(s): ______________________________

ICD-10-CM Code(s): ______________________________

ICD-9-CM Code(s): ______________________________

Abstracting Questions

1. The bone fragments were submitted in formalin. What is formalin? ______________________________

Case 13-6: Endometrial Curettage

LOCATION: Outpatient, Hospital

PATIENT: Kimberly Lakeland

ATTENDING PHYSICIAN: Ira Avila, MD

SURGEON: Ira Avila, MD

PATHOLOGIST: Grey Lonewolf, MD

CLINICAL HISTORY: Dysfunctional uterine bleeding. Recent false-positive serum HCG, last delivery 1 year ago.

SPECIMEN RECEIVED: Endometrial curettings.

GROSS DESCRIPTION: Submitted in formalin and labeled with patient's name and "endometrial curettings" are multiple fragments of tan-brown tissue measuring approximately 3 cc in aggregate. Submitted in toto.

MICROSCOPIC DIAGNOSIS: The slide shows multiple fragments of endometrial tissue featuring an overall normal gland-to-stroma ratio. The glands are somewhat irregular and coiled, and the majority of glands feature subnuclear vacuoles. The stroma is mildly to moderately edematous and bland.

DIAGNOSIS: Uterus, endometrium, curettage; early secretory phase endometrium.

CPT Code(s): ______________________________

ICD-10-CM Code(s): ______________________________

ICD-9-CM Code(s): ______________________________

Abstracting Questions

1. What is a serum HCG? ______________________________

Case 13-7: Cerebral Hematoma

LOCATION: Inpatient, Hospital

PATIENT: Daniel Smithson

ATTENDING PHYSICIAN: Timothy Pleasant, MD

SURGEON: Timothy Pleasant, MD

PATHOLOGIST: Grey Lonewolf, MD

CLINICAL HISTORY: Nontraumatic cerebral bleeding.

SPECIMEN RECEIVED: Cerebral hematoma.

GROSS DESCRIPTION: Submitted in formalin and labeled with the patient's name and "cerebral hematoma" are fragments of reddish brown blood clot measuring approximately 4.5 × 3.5 × 1.5 cm in aggregate. Representative fragments are submitted in one cassette.

MICROSCOPIC DIAGNOSIS: Sections show fragments of fresh blood clot and a single fragment of brain parenchyma featuring intact cortex and underlying white matter and mild-to-moderate edema. No neoplasm is identified.

DIAGNOSIS: Cerebral hematoma, evacuation: Recent blood clot and benign brain parenchyma.

CPT Code(s): ____________________

ICD-10-CM Code(s): ____________________

ICD-9-CM Code(s): ____________________

Abstracting Questions

1. How many cassettes were submitted? ____________________

Case 13-8: Necrotic Fascia

LOCATION: Outpatient, Hospital

PATIENT: Gary Ivy

ATTENDING PHYSICIAN: Ira Avila, MD

SURGEON: Ira Avila, MD

PATHOLOGIST: Grey Lonewolf, MD

CLINICAL HISTORY: Boil left groin; diabetes.

SPECIMEN RECEIVED: Necrotic fascia left groin and leg (anterior and posterior).

GROSS DESCRIPTION: The specimen is labeled with the patient's name and "fascia left groin and leg," and consists of multiple segments of skin and soft tissue measuring up to 30 cm in greatest dimension. The skin is unremarkable, with soft tissue being hemorrhagic and friable and foul smelling.

MICROSCOPIC DIAGNOSIS: Sections of skin and soft tissue show coagulative necrosis with neutrophilic exudate.

DIAGNOSIS: Skin and soft tissue, left groin and leg, anterior and posterior showing coagulative necrosis and acute inflammation.

CPT Code(s): ____________________

ICD-10-CM Code(s): ____________________

ICD-9-CM Code(s): ____________________

Abstracting Questions

1. Was the tissue in this report soft tissue? ____________________
2. What is meant by soft tissue? ____________________

Case 13-9: Myxoma

LOCATION: Inpatient, Hospital

PATIENT: Beverly Hill

ATTENDING PHYSICIAN: Gary Sanchez, MD

SURGEON: Gary Sanchez, MD

PATHOLOGIST: Grey Lonewolf, MD

CLINICAL HISTORY: Mass left atrium.

SPECIMEN RECEIVED: Myxoma—left atrium with FS.

GROSS DESCRIPTION: The specimen is labeled with the patient's name and "left atrial myxoma," and consists of a 4 × 2 × 2 cm ovoid mass with a partially calcified hemorrhagic white-tan tissue.

INTRAOPERATIVE FROZEN SECTION DIAGNOSIS: Myxoma, per Dr. Lonewolf.

MICROSCOPIC DIAGNOSIS: Sections show a well-circumscribed mass consisting of fibromyxoid tissue showing numerous vascular channels. Areas of superficial ulceration and chronic inflammatory infiltrate are noted. Areas of calcification are also present.

DIAGNOSIS: Myxoma, benign, left atrium.

CPT Code(s): ______________________________

ICD-10-CM Code(s): ______________________________

ICD-9-CM Code(s): ______________________________

Abstracting Questions

1. The Specimen Received section indicates "FS." What does FS stand for? ______________________________
2. Was the intraoperative FS reported separately? ______________________________

Case 13-10: Soleus Muscle

LOCATION: Outpatient, Hospital

PATIENT: Darrin Hull

ATTENDING PHYSICIAN: Ira Avila, MD

SURGEON: Ira Avila, MD

PATHOLOGIST: Grey Lonewolf, MD

CLINICAL HISTORY: Necrotic soleus muscle right leg.

SPECIMEN RECEIVED: Soleus muscle right leg.

GROSS DESCRIPTION: Submitted in formalin and labeled with the patient's name and "soleus muscle right leg" are multiple irregular fragments of tan, gray, and brown soft tissue measuring 8 × 8 × 2.5 cm in aggregate. Multiple representative fragments are submitted in four cassettes.

MICROSCOPIC DIAGNOSIS: The slides show multiple sections of skeletal muscle showing severe coagulative and liquefactive necrosis. Patchy neutrophilic infiltrates are present within the necrotic tissue.

DIAGNOSIS: Soft tissue, soleus muscle, right leg, debridement; soft necrosis and patchy acute inflammation, skeletal muscle, fragments of.

CPT Code(s): ____________________

ICD-10-CM Code(s): ____________________

ICD-9-CM Code(s): ____________________

Abstracting Questions

1. How many cassettes were submitted? ____________________

Chapter 14

Pediatrics, Neonatology, and Adolescent Medicine

Make sure to check evolve learning system for the latest content updates

Case 14-1: Well-Child Check

CLINIC NOTE

LOCATION: Outpatient, Hospital

PATIENT: Bradley Wellingstone

PHYSICIAN: Rolando Ortez, MD

SUBJECTIVE: This is a 3-week-old former 32-week gestational male infant who was in RNICU from birth. He did have some mild respiratory difficulties, oxygen requirements that resolved without further sequelae. He was also there for sepsis and feeding difficulties as well as apnea. He was discharged home on caffeine citrate, home apnea monitoring. He did return 2 days ago to get his first dose of Synagis. He is here for general checkup otherwise.

OBJECTIVE: He is on 24-calorie Enfamil and is taking that well without difficulty, taking almost 2 ounces at feeding; urinating and stool schedule is normal. No other complaints from his mother.

ASSESSMENT: On exam, alert, in no distress, and afebrile. His weight is up to 2341 grams, which is up 150 grams. Fontanelle, eyes, ears, nose, and pharynx are clear. Neck is supple. Lungs are clear to auscultation. Heart is regular rate and rhythm without murmur. Abdomen benign. Extremities: Full range of motion. No hip abnormalities. Skin is without rash. Neurologic exam without defect.

IMPRESSION: Thriving former 32-weeker. Now 3 weeks old.

PLAN: Anticipatory guidance discussed. We talked about feeding issues, accident prevention, car seat use, sleeping position on the side or the back. We will see them back in 1 month for his next Synagis dose as well as a recheck. We will have him on caffeine citrate 10 mg/day along with home apnea monitoring with plans to stop the caffeine in 1 month. With any problems, they need to give us a call or come back in sooner for re-evaluation.

CPT Code(s): ______________________________

ICD-10-CM Code(s): ______________________________

ICD-9-CM Code(s): ______________________________

Abstracting Questions

1. From what CPT section would a code be located to report this? ______________________
2. From what CPT subcategory would this service be reported? ______________________
3. Was the patient a new or established patient with the provider? ______________________
4. Does the age of the patient affect code assignment? ______________________
5. What type of diagnosis code was reported? ______________________

Case 14-2: NICU Progress Note, Prematurity with Respiratory Difficulty

This is the initial service by Dr. Ortez for this patient.

LOCATION: Inpatient, Hospital

PATIENT: Sorrento Hernandez

PHYSICIAN: Rolando Ortez, MD

CHIEF COMPLAINT: Prematurity with respiratory difficulty.

HISTORY: This is a 30 weeks, 2 days' gestation female infant with birth weight of 1808 grams. Mom is a 26-year-old gravida 2, now para 2 mom. Her blood type is O positive, antibody negative, RPR nonreactive, rubella immune, hepatitis B surface antigen negative, HIV negative, GC negative, chlamydia negative, Group B Strep status unknown. Mom's MSAFP was elevated at 14.2 with a 1:180 risk for Down syndrome. No neural tube defect. No amniocentesis performed. She was on prenatal vitamins.

First pregnancy went to 35 weeks without complications. He is doing well at 10 years of age; however, he does have Noonan syndrome.

I did attend the delivery of the baby. Spontaneous cry noted, and Apgar score was 7 at 1 minute, with points off for color, tone, and grimace, and then at 5 minutes, Apgar score of 8 with points off for grimace and tone. The infant was then brought back to the NICU for further management.

Baby's face does look somewhat dysmorphic with concerns for Noonan syndrome; very small posterior pharyngeal space was noted with difficult intubation, and after several attempts, the anesthesiology department was called and the infant was intubated. Throughout the intubation attempts, standard procedure was followed and the baby tolerated the attempts very well. The intubation was performed because of concerns of hypoventilation noted on exam with decreased breath sounds bilaterally as well as increased work of breathing.

Umbilical artery catheter was also placed without difficulty. First blood sugar did come back at 23, a peripheral IV was placed promptly, and 2 cc/kilo of D10 was given along with placing the infant on D10 at 80 cc/kilo. Second blood sugar has come back elevated.

Chest x-ray is obtained as well as abdominal films and shows good placement of the UAC at T7, and the endotracheal tube is also in good placement and is a 3.02. The OG has been advanced. The lung fields do show significant granularity present. No pneumothorax, no cardiomegaly. Blood gas is 7.32, PCO_2 of 50, PO_2 of 100 and that is on a setting of 22/4, rate of 60% and 80% FIO_2.

PHYSICAL EXAMINATION: Currently is intubated, her weight is 1808 grams. OFC is 30.5 cm, length is 39.4 cm. Heart rate is in the 130s to 140s. Respiratory rate is at 60 on the ventilator. O_2 sat is in the mid 90s. Blood pressure is right arm, 67/34 with a mean of 46, right leg 67/32 with a mean of 44.

Mild splitting of the cranial sutures is noted along with open posterior and anterior fontanel. Red reflex ×2. Eyes appear to have hypertelorism present and questionable epicanthal folds along with some down-slanting palpebral fissures. Ears appear to be low set and posteriorly rotated. Palate is intact. There is a small retropharyngeal space. Clavicles are intact. I do not appreciate any webbing on the neck. Nipples, questionable, mildly wide spaced. Lungs at this time are clear to auscultation. She has good symmetric aeration; minimal chest rise noted. Prior to that, lungs were remarkable for decreased aeration with crackles. Heart is regular rate and rhythm, no murmurs noted. Femoral pulses palpable, cap refill less than 2 seconds. Abdomen is without hepatosplenomegaly, three-vessel cord. Genitourinary: Normal female. Extremities: Adequate range of motion, no contractures or hip abnormalities noted. Skin is ruddy in complexion. Neurologic Exam: Hypotonia diffusely.

Developmental assessment: No breast buds, soft pinna with minimal recoil, no creases on the feet, consistent with a 30-week preterm infant.

IMPRESSION
1. Premature female infant.
2. Respiratory distress consistent with hyaline membrane disease as well as a component of hypoventilation secondary to maternal elevated magnesium.
3. Observation for sepsis.
4. Maternal hypermagnesemia with elevated magnesium in the infant as well.
5. Family history of Noonan syndrome in an older brother.

PLAN: Admission to the NICU. Intubation has been performed, and she is on mechanical ventilation. Will go ahead with the surfactant therapy per protocol, close cardiorespiratory monitoring and monitoring of blood gases and chest x-rays. NPO status, and she will be on D10 with 0.94 mEq of calcium gluconate added to run at 80 cc/kilo/day. Ampicillin and gentamicin administered per protocol. Blood cultures have been obtained as well as a CBC, magnesium level, and further glucose monitoring. She will also need chromosomal testing, and that will be drawn in the near future. Also, head ultrasound at 6 days of life will need to be performed. I have not talked with the mother. Her condition has deteriorated post cesarean section and is not available at this time. I have talked in detail with the father in regard to the above, including possibility of further deterioration prompting transfer to another facility. All his questions have been addressed.

CPT Code(s): ______________________________

ICD-10-CM Code(s): ______________________________

ICD-9-CM Code(s): ______________________________

Abstracting Questions

1. Was this the initial or subsequent visit? ______________________________
2. Does the age of the patient affect CPT code selection? ______________________________
3. What two factors affect diagnosis code assignment? ______________________________

Case 14-3: Progress Note, Ventilator Assist

This is a subsequent hospital visit by Dr. Ortez for this patient.

LOCATION: Inpatient, Hospital

PATIENT: Manuel Sanchez

PHYSICIAN: Rolando Ortez, MD

SUBJECTIVE: This baby boy is slightly under 24 hours.

OBJECTIVE: Weight today is 1.851 kg (increased 43 grams over birth weight). OFC is 30.5 cm (unchanged). Intake and output from yesterday do appear adequate, although it was less than 24 hours. He has had no stool since birth. Vital signs reveal his temperature to be acceptable while being maintained on an open radiant warmer. Heart rate is generally in the 110s–140s. Respiratory rate is generally equal to the IMV (60). Mean blood pressures had decreased last night to the low 30s but are now in the low to mid 40s while on dopamine infusion.

PHYSICAL EXAMINATION: In general, he is pink concurrent with ventilator setting. He does appear slightly dysmorphic with eyes wide set and slightly down-slanting palpebral fissures. Ears appear low set and posteriorly rotated. Endotracheal tube is in place. Chest reveals symmetric expansion and the lungs are clear to auscultation on current ventilator settings. Cardiac exam reveals a regular rate without murmur or click. Peripheral pulses are 2+ and symmetric. Abdominal exam reveals an umbilical arterial catheter in place. Liver is palpable 1 cm below the right costal margin. No splenomegaly or masses were noted. Genital examination reveals normal male, testes are not palpable. Extremity examination reveals no fixed decreased range of motion, deformity, or joint abnormality. Neurologic exam reveals diffuse hypotonia. No focal deficits are appreciated.

CURRENT MEDICATIONS
1. Ampicillin 90.4 mg IV q12h.
2. Gentamicin 5.4 mg IV 1q18h.
3. Morphine sulfate 0.18 mg IV q6h and q1h p.r.n.
4. Dopamine 5 mcg/kg/min.
5. Vecuronium 0.18 mg IV q1-2h p.r.n.

LABORATORY STUDIES: Last arterial blood gas was obtained on ventilator settings of IMV 60, pressure 22/4, and FIO_2 0.53 and revealed pH 7.3, PCO_2 46.6, PO_2 52.7, and bicarbonate 22.7. Chemistry panel this morning revealed sodium 123, potassium 5.7, chloride 93, glucose 66, BUN 12, creatinine 0.9, calcium 7.3, magnesium 5.4, phosphorus 6.8, bilirubin 4.4, alkaline phosphatase 200, ALT 14, AST 38, albumin 1.7, and total protein 3.6. Electrolytes were repeated and were unchanged. CBC with differential this morning revealed a white count of 8230 with 6 bands, 45 neutrophils, 31 lymphocytes, 7 monocytes, and 7 eosinophils. Platelet count was 98,000. Chest x-ray continues to show significant evidence of hyaline membrane disease.

IMPRESSIONS/RECOMMENDATIONS
1. Less than 24-hour-old infant who was born at 30 weeks' gestation. Based on clinical examination, he may have Noonan syndrome.
2. Respiratory: He has evidence of hyaline membrane disease with respiratory failure. He had received two doses of surfactant and will receive a third dose soon. We will adjust his ventilator setting based on serial clinical examinations, pulse oximetry, arterial blood gas determinations, and chest x-rays. Will continue sedation and paralysis at this time. I would recommend a short course of steroids because of the intubation attempts when he is extubated.

3. Cardiovascular: Cardiovascular status is acceptable at this time while on dopamine at 5 mcg/kg/min. Blood pressure has improved on inotropic support. I do not hear a murmur at this time. He may require echocardiography to evaluate for PDA depending on his clinical course.
4. Gastrointestinal: Abdominal exam remains benign. He is NPO. He has mild hyperbilirubinemia, and mom is noted to have O positive blood and Rh. We are going to obtain a direct antibody test. Will follow with serial bilirubin determinations.
5. Hematologic: He has developed a mild thrombocytopenia; will monitor.
6. Infectious Disease: Blood culture remains negative; he is on ampicillin and gentamicin. We will check closely.
7. Neurologic: Exam remains acceptable given his extreme prematurity. He will require screening intracranial ultrasounds and long-term neurodevelopmental follow-up.
8. Renal/Metabolic: Urine output remains adequate at this time. Metabolic parameters were acceptable. Will monitor closely.
9. Fluid/Electrolytes/Nutrition: He has gained some weight since birth. Multiple electrolyte dysfunctions are noted. This is partially due to dilution. We have restricted fluid somewhat and added various electrolytes/minerals to his TPN. We will monitor with serial chemistry panels.
10. Apnea/Bradycardia: None since birth.
11. Health Care Maintenance: None yet.

SOCIAL HISTORY: Mom and dad have been kept up to date with regard to their son's condition. Their questions have been answered, and they are in agreement with the outlined management plan.

CPT Code(s): ______________________________

ICD-10-CM Code(s): ______________________________

ICD-9-CM Code(s): ______________________________

Abstracting Questions

1. For CPT code assignment, would this be an initial or subsequent service? ______________________

Case 14-4: NICU Progress Note, Ventilator Assist

Dr. Ortez has been following this infant since birth.

LOCATION: Inpatient, Hospital

PATIENT: Loren Black

ATTENDING PHYSICIAN: Rolando Ortez, MD

SUBJECTIVE: Baby is currently 2 days old, slightly under 48 hours.

OBJECTIVE: Weight today is 1716 kg (decreased by 135 grams). He is down 5.1% of his weight since birth. OFC is 30 cm (decreased 0.5 cm). Intake yesterday was 152 cc, 82 cc/kg/day. Output was 170 cc, 3.8 cc/kg/hour. He has had no stools since birth. Vital signs reveal his temperature to be acceptable while on an open, radiant warmer. Heart rate is generally in the 110s–120s. Respiratory rate has generally been equal to the IMV (60). Mean blood pressures have generally been in the 40s–50s. Oxygen saturations have remained in the high 90s.

PHYSICAL EXAMINATION: In general, he is pink, on current ventilator settings. He does have slightly dysmorphic features with wide-set eyes and slightly down-slanting palpebral fissures. Ears are low set and posteriorly rotated. Endotracheal tube was in place. Neck was without masses. Chest reveals symmetric expansion and lungs are clear to auscultation on current ventilator settings. Cardiac Exam: Regular rate without murmur or click. Peripheral pulses are 2+ and symmetric. Abdominal Exam: UAC in place. Liver is palpable 1 cm below the right costal margin. No splenomegaly or masses were noted. Genital Exam: Normal male. Testes are not palpable. Extremity Exam: No fixed decreased range of motion, deformity, or joint abnormality. Neurologic Exam: Mild, diffuse hypotonia. No focal deficits are appreciated.

CURRENT MEDICATIONS
1. Ampicillin 90.4 mg IV q12h.
2. Gentamicin 5.4 mg IV q18h.
3. Morphine sulfate 0.18 mg IV q6h and q1h p.r.n.
4. Dopamine 5 mcg/kg/min.
5. Vecuronium 0.18 mg IV q1-2h p.r.n.

LABORATORY STUDIES: Last arterial blood gas was obtained on ventilator setting of IMV 60, pressures of 24/4, and FIO_2 of 0.5 revealed pH 7.27, PCO_2 51.1, PO_2 66.5, and bicarbonate 22.5. Chemistry panel this morning reveals sodium of 134, potassium of 4.9, chloride of 102, glucose of 111, BUN of 18, creatinine of 1.0, calcium of 7.5, magnesium of 3.8, phosphorus of 7.7, bilirubin of 7.8. CBC reveals a white count of 6190. Platelet count was 98,000. Chest x-ray continues to show significant evidence of hyaline membrane disease. Endotracheal tube is near the carina and has been withdrawn somewhat.

IMPRESSION/RECOMMENDATIONS
1. Two-day-old infant who was born at 30 weeks' gestation. He does have clinical features suggestive of Noonan syndrome.
2. Respiratory: Continues to show evidence of hyaline membrane disease with respiratory failure. He has received three doses of surfactant therapy. He does have echocardiographic evidence of PDA, and we will be treating this at this time. We will attempt to decrease his ventilator settings based on serial clinical examination, pulse oximetry, arterial blood gas determinations, and chest x-ray.
3. Cardiovascular: Status is acceptable at this time while on dopamine at 5 mcg/kg/min. Echocardiogram shows a patent ductus arteriosis. There also appears to be a slight

abnormality to the pulmonary valve, which could be associated with his possible Noonan syndrome. He is going to receive indomethacin therapy.

4. Gastrointestinal: Abdominal exam remains benign. He is NPO. He does have mild hyperbilirubinemia. Direct antibody test was negative. We will begin phototherapy at this time.
5. Hematologic: Serial CBCs have been acceptable except for mild thrombocytopenia. We will continue to monitor, especially in light of the indomethacin therapy. He has not required any blood product transfusions since birth.
6. Infectious Disease: Blood culture remains negative at this time. We have discontinued his gentamicin, and he is being placed on cefotaxime because of the indomethacin.
7. Neurologic: Exam remains acceptable given his extreme prematurity. He will require screening intracranial ultrasound and long-term neurodevelopmental follow-up.
8. Renal/Metabolic: Urine output remains adequate and renal function studies are acceptable. Previous metabolic parameters are acceptable. We will repeat in the morning.
9. Fluids/Electrolytes/Nutrition: Weight loss is acceptable and electrolytes are in the more normal range today. We will adjust his TPN accordingly.
10. Apnea/Bradycardia: None since birth.
11. Health Care Maintenance: None yet.

SOCIAL HISTORY: Mom and dad are being kept up to date with regard to the patient's condition. Their questions have been answered, and they are in agreement with the outlined management plan.

CPT Code(s): ______________________________

ICD-10-CM Code(s): ______________________________

ICD-9-CM Code(s): ______________________________

Abstracting Questions

1. The surfactant therapy was given for which diagnosis? ______________________________
2. What does PDA mean? ______________________________

Case 14-5: Circumcision

LOCATION: Inpatient, Hospital

PATIENT: Samuel Hill

ATTENDING PHYSICIAN: Rolando Ortez, MD

SURGEON: Rolando Ortez, MD

PROCEDURE: Circumcision.

PREOPERATIVE DIAGNOSIS: Phimosis and parental request for circumcision.

POSTOPERATIVE DIAGNOSIS: Same.

INDICATIONS FOR PROCEDURE: This is a 2-month-old male who was born extremely premature at 30 weeks' gestation. He is nearing the end of his hospitalization, and parents have requested a circumcision. Potential benefits, risks, and complications of the circumcision, including lidocaine anesthesia, were reviewed with the family. Their questions were answered, and they are in agreement with the outlined plan.

PROCEDURE: The baby was appropriately restrained on the circumcision board. The penis and groin area were cleansed thoroughly with Betadine. One-percent lidocaine without epinephrine was injected at the 10-o'clock and 2-o'clock positions with good anesthetic result. In addition, he received oral glucose water. Circumcision was performed using 1.1-cm Gomco clamp with standard technique. After completion of the circumcision, sterile Vaseline gauze was applied.

COMPLICATIONS: No immediate complications were noted.

CPT Code(s): ____________________

ICD-10-CM Code(s): ____________________

ICD-9-CM Code(s): ____________________

Abstracting Questions

1. Does the method of circumcision affect CPT code selection? ____________________
2. Which modifier may be reported with the CPT code 54150 when the procedure is performed without a dorsal penile or ring block? ____________________
3. What modifier is never reported with 54150? ____________________
4. Does the age of the patient affect code selection for a circumcision? ____________________

Case 14-6: Newborn Report

Report the newborn service for this single, 8-pound 2-ounce newborn delivered on October 1.

LOCATION: Inpatient, Hospital

PATIENT: Robert Stilwell

ATTENDING PHYSICIAN: Rolando Ortez, MD

NEWBORN EXAM RECORD

ADMISSION EXAM Date: 10/1
DISCHARGE EXAM Date: 10/5

	Normal	Abnormal		Normal	Abnormal	
Head/Fontanels		X	1-cm area between fontanels	X		Head healing well
Eyes	X			X		
Ears/Nose/Throat		X			X	
Heart	X			X		
Lungs	X			X		
Abdomen	X			X		
Trunk/Spine	X			X		
Anus	X			X		
Genitalia	X			X		
Negative Barlow Test		X			X	
Negative Ortolani Test		X			X	
Extremities/Clavicles		X			X	
Skin	X			X		
Neurlogical/Tone		X			X	

PROGRESS NOTES:

10/2 Exam on 1 x top of head, which is clean and dry. Color good. Wt down 2.5%. Nursing poorly. GJH	
10/3 Exam: Head healing well. Color good. Nursing better. Wt down 5%. Circumcised per parent request. GJH	
10/4 Exam: Wt down 6%. Nursing poorly. Color good. GJH	
10/5 Exam: Wt down 8%. Nursing poorly. Discharge from the hospital, and I will see on Monday in the office. GJH	
	Hearing Exam: Passed AZ

CPT Code(s): ______________________________

ICD-10-CM Code(s): ______________________________

ICD-9-CM Code(s): ______________________________

Abstracting Questions

1. How many services were reported? ______________________________
2. Five of the services are from what CPT section? ______________________________
3. What is the non-E/M service? ______________________________
4. Will a modifier be required for the E/M service on 10/3? ______________________________
5. What type of diagnosis code was assigned? ______________________________

Chapter 15
Diagnostic Radiology

Make sure to check evolve learning system for the latest content updates

Case 15-1: CT of Brain

RADIOLOGY REPORT

LOCATION: Outpatient, Hospital

PATIENT: Sally Church

ORDERING PHYSICIAN: Timothy L. Pleasant, MD

ATTENDING/ADMIT PHYSICIAN: Timothy L. Pleasant, MD

RADIOLOGIST: Morton Monson, MD

PERSONAL PHYSICIAN: Ronald Green, MD

EXAMINATION: CT of the brain.

CLINICAL SYMPTOMS: Headache, enlarged left pupil.

COMPUTED TOMOGRAPHIC EXAMINATION OF BRAIN: Performed without contrast material. This is an emergency procedure.

There is blood within the suprasellar cistern, more so on the left than the right. Blood extends slightly anteriorly along the anterior cerebral arteries and slightly laterally along the proximal portion of the middle cerebral arteries. On image 6, there does appear to be a 7- to 8-mm collection of increased density. This may well be clotted blood. It might also be an aneurysm. A small amount of blood is also present in the cisterna ambiens, making that cistern slightly less visualized.

There is a small amount of blood within the third ventricle and small amounts of blood in the posterior portions of the lateral ventricles. The lateral ventricles show mild dilation. Several cerebral sulci can be visualized at the vertex.

IMPRESSION: Headache and pupil dilatation due to acute nontraumatic subarachnoid hemorrhage with blood collected mainly anteriorly in relation to the suprasellar cistern.

CPT Code(s): ______________________________

ICD-10-CM Code(s): ______________________________

ICD-9-CM Code(s): ______________________________

Abstracting Questions

1. What body area was evaluated? ______________________________
2. Was contrast material used? ______________________________
3. What CPT modifier was appended to the code used to report this service? ______________________________

Case 15-2: X-Ray, Chest

RADIOLOGY REPORT

LOCATION: Outpatient, Hospital

PATIENT: Sue Chang

ORDERING PHYSICIAN: Gregory Dawson, MD

ATTENDING/ADMIT PHYSICIAN: Gregory Dawson, MD

RADIOLOGIST: Morton Monson, MD

PERSONAL PHYSICIAN: Ronald Green, MD

EXAMINATION: X-ray, chest

CLINICAL SYMPTOMS: Sounds in the chest.

TWO X-RAY VIEWS OF CHEST: Comparison is made with the chest films of August 13. Heart size: Upper limits of normal and unchanged. Pulmonary vascularity is borderline increased and stable. Left pleural effusion has decreased in size. Area of infiltrate and/or atelectasis in the left mid and lower lung has decreased somewhat in the left perihilar region. Nodular infiltrate and/or atelectasis in the right midlung is not significantly changed. Area of infiltrate and/or atelectasis in the right infrahilar region is small and unchanged. Hypertrophic changes, thoracic spine.

CPT Code(s): ______________________________

ICD-10-CM Code(s): ______________________________

ICD-9-CM Code(s): ______________________________

Abstracting Questions

1. How many views were taken? ______________________________
2. Was the review of the previous films reported separately? ______________________________

Case 15-3: Cranial CT

RADIOLOGY REPORT

LOCATION: Inpatient, Hospital

PATIENT: Bill Arnold

ORDERING PHYSICIAN: Timothy L. Pleasant, MD

ATTENDING/ADMIT PHYSICIAN: Timothy L. Pleasant, MD

RADIOLOGIST: Morton Monson, MD

PERSONAL PHYSICIAN: Ronald Green, MD

EXAMINATION: Cranial CT.

CLINICAL SYMPTOMS: Altered mental status.

TECHNIQUE: Axial noncontrast CT scan of the head.

INTERPRETATION: There is diffuse mild enlargement of the sulci and ventricles. Periventricular diminished density is present bilaterally and is prominent near the trigones of the lateral ventricles. There is a 1-mm high-density area seen on image 10 in the left posterior temporal occipital region.

In the posterior fossa the fourth ventricle is normal in position. Mildly prominent cerebellar folia are present.

No abnormalities of the orbits, paranasal sinuses, or temporal bone can be seen.

There is a small amount of calcification in the paraclinoid and carotid arteries.

CONCLUSIONS
1. Mild diffuse cerebral atrophy.
2. Periventricular changes consistent with age-related ischemic change.
3. Tiny calcification in the left posterior temporal occipital region. Finding is nonspecific and could reflect previous granulomatous calcification, intraluminal calcification, Pantopaque, or calcification in a lesion. Recommend clinical correlation and cranial MRI if appropriate.
4. Vascular calcifications are present.

CPT Code(s): ______________________

ICD-10-CM Code(s): ______________________

ICD-9-CM Code(s): ______________________

Abstracting Questions

1. What was the clinical symptom that prompted this CT? ______________________
2. Sulci were referred to in the Interpretation section. What are sulci? ______________________

Case 15-4: X-Ray, Chest

RADIOLOGY REPORT

LOCATION: Outpatient, Hospital

PATIENT: Melissa Wellington

ORDERING PHYSICIAN: Ronald Green, MD

ATTENDING/ADMIT PHYSICIAN: Ronald Green, MD

RADIOLOGIST: Morton Monson, MD

PERSONAL PHYSICIAN: Ronald Green, MD

EXAMINATION: X-ray, chest.

CLINICAL SYMPTOMS: Follow-up of pneumonia.

PA AND LATERAL CHEST X-RAY: Comparison is made with the previous study of July 29.

There is evidence of antecedent midline sternotomy. The heart continues to be mildly prominent. Bibasilar effusions are noted. There is some consolidation seen in the right mainstem bronchus, which may represent atelectasis or loculated fluid. This, of course, will need to be followed to ensure that it resolves. The upper lung fields are relatively clearer than seen on the previous study. Endotracheal tube and nasogastric tube have been removed. Bipolar endocardiac pacing device is unchanged in position. The lung fields are somewhat hyperinflated. The aorta is arteriosclerotic. Degenerative changes are seen through the dorsal spine.

CONCLUSIONS

1. Ventilation within the lung fields has improved when compared with the previous study. There appear to be bibasilar effusions, more prominent on the right. There is also some focal consolidation within the right medial lower lobe just under the right mainstem bronchus. This is a somewhat lobular consolidation, and I suspect this may be localized fluid or atelectasis. This, of course, will need to be followed closely to ensure that it resolves. If not, then CT may be necessary.
2. Mild cardiomegaly with central vascularity now at the upper norm.
3. Bipolar endocardiac pacing device, unchanged in position.
4. Aortic arteriosclerotic vascular disease.
5. Probable underlying chronic obstructive pulmonary disease.
6. Degenerative changes of the dorsal spine.
7. Interim removal of nasogastric tube when compared with the prior study.

CPT Code(s): ______________________________

ICD-10-CM Code(s): ______________________________

ICD-9-CM Code(s): ______________________________

Abstracting Questions

1. What does point 3 in the Conclusion section of the report refer to? ______________________
2. Not only does this patient have pneumonia, she also was noted to probably have this type of chronic pulmonary disease. What was this "probable" disease? ______________________

Case 15-5: CT of Abdomen and Pelvis

RADIOLOGY REPORT

LOCATION: Outpatient, Clinic

PATIENT: Max Rey

ORDERING PHYSICIAN: Ronald Green, MD

ATTENDING/ADMIT PHYSICIAN: Ronald Green, MD

RADIOLOGIST: Morton Monson, MD

PERSONAL PHYSICIAN: Ronald Green, MD

EXAMINATION: CT of abdomen and pelvis.

CLINICAL SYMPTOMS: Ascites.

TECHNIQUE: CT of the abdomen and pelvis was performed without oral or IV contrast material per physician request. No previous CT scans for comparison.

FINDINGS: No ascites. Moderate-size right pleural effusion. Small left pleural effusion. Associated compressive atelectasis with these effusions. Pacemaker leads in place. Negative adrenal glands. No definite focal hepatic or splenic lesions. Marked distention of the stomach with air-fluid level. Vague, approximately 2-cm, low-density lesion in the midportion of the left kidney may represent a cyst. Sigmoid diverticulosis. No free air or free fluid. A Foley catheter was placed within the bladder. Prostatic enlargement. Small amount of air within the bladder lumen likely due to recent catheterization. Vascular calcification. Adrenal glands are negative. Grossly negative pancreas. Mild soft tissue stranding about both kidneys is of uncertain etiology and clinical significance.

CPT Code(s): ____________________

ICD-10-CM Code(s): ____________________

ICD-9-CM Code(s): ____________________

Abstracting Questions

1. Define ascites. ____________________
2. Although not reported with a diagnosis code, the radiologist noted that the patient had this located in the left kidney. ____________________
3. Why would the diagnosis in question 2 not be reported? ____________________

Case 15-6: Gallbladder Ultrasound

RADIOLOGY REPORT

LOCATION: Outpatient, Hospital

PATIENT: Dan Diel

ORDERING PHYSICIAN: Daniel G. Olanka, MD

ATTENDING/ADMIT PHYSICIAN: Daniel G. Olanka, MD

RADIOLOGIST: Morton Monson, MD

PERSONAL PHYSICIAN: Ronald Green, MD

EXAMINATION: Gallbladder ultrasound.

CLINICAL SYMPTOMS: Increased bilirubin.

GALLBLADDER ULTRASOUND: Examination was technically difficult with some limitations due to overlying leads. Large right pleural effusion identified. Gallbladder is visualized. No obvious gallstones or gallbladder wall thickening. Only short portions of the common hepatic duct and common bile duct are visualized. Common hepatic duct measures 3.6 mm, and common bile duct measures 5.2 mm. These values are within normal limits. There is limited assessment of the liver, which is grossly unremarkable.

IMPRESSION: Gallbladder ultrasound with limitations as discussed above. Grossly unremarkable sonographic appearance of the gallbladder. No obvious dilatation of the common duct. Large right pleural effusion identified.

CPT Code(s): ______________________________

ICD-10-CM Code(s): ______________________________

ICD-9-CM Code(s): ______________________________

Abstracting Questions

1. What subcategory within Radiology in the CPT was referenced for assignment of a code for this case?

   ____

2. What body area was evaluated? ______________________________
3. What code range in the CPT was reviewed to select the Ultrasound code? ______________________________
4. What modifier was appended to the CPT code? ______________________________

Case 15-7: Ultrasound, Kidneys

RADIOLOGY REPORT

LOCATION: Outpatient, Hospital

PATIENT: Eldon Philip

ORDERING PHYSICIAN: Ira Avila, MD

ATTENDING/ADMIT PHYSICIAN: Ira Avila, MD

RADIOLOGIST: Morton Monson, MD

PERSONAL PHYSICIAN: Ronald Green, MD

EXAMINATION: Ultrasound of the kidneys.

CLINICAL SYMPTOMS: Elevated BUN.

ULTRASOUND OF KIDNEYS: We are also asked to look at the urinary bladder and calculate residual volume postvoid. Right kidney is 11.3 × 5.5 × 5.8 cm. The renal parenchymal thickness is within normal limits for age grouping. No cystic or solid mass is seen. No dilated collecting system is present to suggest obstruction.

The left kidney is 11.9 × 5.9 × 6.9 cm. Again, no cystic or solid mass or dilated collecting system is seen.

Both kidneys were difficult to image due to large body habitus. We have, however, excluded obstruction and gross mass lesion.

The urinary bladder shows smooth contour. Postvoid residual volume of the urinary bladder is estimated at 59 cc.

IMPRESSION: Normal ultrasound of kidneys and bladder.

CPT Code(s): ____________________

ICD-10-CM Code(s): ____________________

ICD-9-CM Code(s): ____________________

Abstracting Questions

1. Why did the radiologist have difficulty imaging on the kidneys? ____________________
2. Did the ultrasound provide a more definitive diagnosis? ____________________

Case 15-8: Catheter Placement

OPERATIVE REPORT

LOCATION: Inpatient, Hospital

PATIENT: Benito Castro

ORDERING PHYSICIAN: Gregory Dawson, MD

ATTENDING/ADMIT PHYSICIAN: Gregory Dawson, MD

RADIOLOGIST: Morton Monson, MD

PERSONAL PHYSICIAN: Ronald Green, MD

EXAMINATION: Placement of a tunneled hemodialysis catheter.

CLINICAL SYMPTOMS: End-stage renal disease.

PLACEMENT OF TUNNELED #14.5 FRENCH HEMODIALYSIS CATHETER: The patient is a 62-year-old male with a history of renal failure. Placement of a tunneled hemodialysis catheter was requested by Dr. Green.

Prior to the start of the study, the procedure was explained to the patient, including the risks, complications, and alternatives. The patient understood and consented to the exam.

The patient was prepped and draped in the usual sterile fashion. An Ioban II (antimicrobial film) was placed on the skin. A 21-gauge micropuncture needle was advanced into the right internal jugular vein in the lower neck region using sterile technique under ultrasound guidance following administration of local anesthesia (1% lidocaine). Utilizing the Microvena kit, a 0.18 stainless steel wire was used to measure the distance from the junction of the right atrium/superior vena cava to the skin site, and the catheter was cut to size. A #5 French straight catheter was advanced into the internal jugular vein. The catheter was then placed to flush.

A small skin incision was placed in the upper chest region. Following administration of local anesthesia (1% lidocaine), a tunnel was obtained between the two skin incisions. A vascular sheath was then placed through the tunnel, and the catheter was advanced through the peel-away sheath.

The #5 French straight catheter was then removed under a Rosen wire, and a #10 French peel-away sheath was placed into the right internal jugular vein. The dilator and wire were then removed, and the end of the peel-away sheath was crimped to avoid blood loss with the patient holding his breath. The tip of the catheter was then advanced through the peel-away sheath with the tip of the junction of the right atrium/superior vena cava. The peel-away sheath was then removed and the catheter was adjusted to obtain a smooth transition. The cuff of the catheter was approximately 1 to 2 cm from the incision site. A single 2–0 Prolene suture was then placed at the catheter insertion site, and three sutures were placed at the lower neck incision site. There was no evidence of bleeding.

Contrast was infused through the single port, which revealed adequate placement.

Post placement chest x-ray did not reveal a pneumothorax.

The patient tolerated the procedure well. The patient denied pain and shortness of breath at termination of the study.

IMPRESSION: Placement of a tunneled #14.5 French hemodialysis catheter through the right internal jugular vein as described above.

CPT Code(s): ____________________

ICD-10-CM Code(s): ____________________

ICD-9-CM Code(s): ____________________

Abstracting Questions

1. Was the catheter inserted by the radiologist? ____________________
2. Was the catheter inserted into the venous or arterial system? ____________________
3. Was the catheter inserted centrally or peripherally? ____________________
4. Was the catheter tunneled? ____________________
5. Was a subcutaneous port/pump inserted? ____________________
6. Does the age of the patient affect CPT code assignment? ____________________
7. Was ultrasound guidance separately reported? ____________________

Case 15-9: Stress Test

RADIOLOGY REPORT

LOCATION: Outpatient, Hospital

PATIENT: Harry Stein

ORDERING PHYSICIAN: James Noonar, MD

ATTENDING/ADMIT PHYSICIAN: James Noonar, MD

RADIOLOGIST: Morton Monson, MD

PERSONAL PHYSICIAN: Ronald Green, MD

EXAMINATION: Adenosine stress test and resting Myoview, left ventricle, with estimate of left ventricular ejection fraction.

CLINICAL SYMPTOMS: Chest pain.

ADENOSINE STRESS AND RESTING MYOVIEW EVALUATION, LEFT VENTRICLE, WITH ESTIMATE OF LEFT VENTRICULAR EJECTION FRACTION: Clinical information states chest pain. This is a patient with known coronary artery disease. The patient has had prior replacement of aortic and mitral valve 3 to 4 years ago by history. The patient has a previous Cardiolite scan from December 24 two years ago that showed "fixed posterior/inferior wall perfusion defect extending into the cardiac apex." On September 12 of this year, the patient was given adenosine challenge under the supervision of Dr. Dawson, who will report on that portion of the evaluation. On September 12, the patient was injected with 27.2 mCi of technetium-99m–tagged tetrofosmin. Views of the left ventricle were then acquired with a SPECT nuclear medicine camera and reformatted into the standard projections. On September 13, the patient was returned to the nuclear medicine department for resting or redistribution scan and injected with 26.2 mCi of technetium-99m–tagged tetrofosmin. Again, views of the left ventricle were acquired with the SPECT nuclear medicine camera and reformatted into standard projections. Comparison of the stress and resting images shows no area to suggest perfusion defect. Nothing to suggest ischemia or infarct is seen. All segments of the left ventricle are perfused.

IMPRESSION
1. Adenosine challenge as the stress. That will be reported by Dr. Dawson.
2. Normal adenosine stress and resting Myoview evaluation, left ventricle. No region suggesting ischemia or infarct.

ADDENDUM: Previously described fixed perfusion defect involving posterior/inferior wall and apex is no longer seen.

Left ventricular ejection fraction estimated at 66%. This is normal. Normal is 50% or greater.

CPT Code(s): ____________________

ICD-10-CM Code(s): ____________________

ICD-9-CM Code(s): ____________________

Abstracting Questions

1. Does use of the SPECT camera affect code assignment? ____________________
2. Were the left ventricular perfusion and ejection fractions reported separately? ____________________

Case 15-10: Ventilation-Perfusion Lung Scan

RADIOLOGY REPORT

LOCATION: Outpatient, Hospital

PATIENT: Les James

ORDERING PHYSICIAN: Gregory Dawson, MD

ATTENDING/ADMIT PHYSICIAN: Gregory Dawson, MD

RADIOLOGIST: Morton Monson, MD

PERSONAL PHYSICIAN: Ronald Green, MD

EXAMINATION: Ventilation-perfusion lung scan.

CLINICAL SYMPTOMS: Pulmonary edema.

VENTILATION-PERFUSION LUNG SCAN: Dose: 2.0 mCi of technetium-99m DTPA via aerosol and 6.0 mCi of technetium-99m MAA IV. No prior studies are available for comparison. I have a portable chest radiograph for correlation. There is significant inhomogeneity and central deposition on the ventilatory scan, suggesting chronic obstructive pulmonary disease. There are areas of decreased ventilation seen bilaterally. There is also some inhomogeneity regarding the perfusion scan. There is marked decreased ventilation and perfusion, right lung base. The patient has right basilar opacity on chest radiograph. Overall probability is indeterminate for pulmonary embolism. No definite segmental ventilation-perfusion mismatches are seen.

IMPRESSION: Indeterminate probability for pulmonary embolism.

CPT Code(s): ____________________

ICD-10-CM Code(s): ____________________

ICD-9-CM Code(s): ____________________

Abstracting Questions

1. What area of the body was studied? ____________________
2. What type of radiological study was performed? ____________________
3. Can the perfusion and ventilation imaging be reported with one code? ____________________
4. Does the aerosol delivery affect code assignment? ____________________

Case 15-11: Head Ultrasound

LOCATION: Inpatient, Hospital

PATIENT: Jason Whittle

ATTENDING PHYSICIAN: Rolando Ortez, MD

CLINICAL SYMPTOMS: Premature, weight 1800 grams.

HEAD ULTRASOUND: Sonographic evaluation of the newborn brain was performed through the anterior fontanel. The study was performed in the coronal and sagittal planes. There is a hyperechoic area seen within the right subependymal region. This measures 0.6 × 0.4 × 0.5 cm. I suspect this is a subependymal hemorrhage. There is also an area within the left intraparenchymal region measuring 0.9 × 1.0 × 1.4 cm. This is a hyperechoic area, which may represent an intraparenchymal hemorrhage on the left parietal/occipital region. There is also question of a small septum cavum pellucidum. This is difficult to state for certain, however.

CONCLUSION
1. What appears to be a right subependymal hemorrhage, as discussed above.
2. Hyperechoic area within the left intraparenchymal region. It may also represent a focal area of hemorrhage measuring 1 cm in greatest diameter.
3. Question of small septum cavum pellucidum as a congenital variation. This is very questionable and difficult to assess for the patient's age. The ventricles themselves do not appear to be grossly dilated.

CPT Code(s): ______________________________

ICD-10-CM Code(s): ______________________________

ICD-9-CM Code(s): ______________________________

Abstracting Questions

1. In what CPT section was the code to report this service located? ______________________________
2. In what CPT category of codes was the code to report this service located? ______________________________

Case 15-12: Abdominal X-Ray, UVC Catheter Placement

LOCATION: Inpatient, Hospital

PATIENT: Samantha Sorette

ATTENDING PHYSICIAN: Rolando Ortez, MD

CLINICAL SYMPTOMS: Umbilical venous catheter placement.

ONE VIEW, ABDOMEN: Single view submitted of the abdomen. Comparison is made with chest/abdomen from earlier this same day. Distal portion of a nasogastric versus OG tube is again seen. There is again umbilical artery catheter, tip to the left of T6. Additional catheter has been placed with tip in the lower pelvis. This presumably reflects the reported UVC line, tip points inferiorly. There is again relatively gasless bowel gas pattern. There is gas-filled bowel loop seen in the left pelvis.

CPT Code(s): ______________________________

ICD-10-CM Code(s): ______________________________

ICD-9-CM Code(s): ______________________________

Abstracting Questions

1. Do the number of views affect code assignment? ______________________________
2. What type of diagnosis code is assigned to report this service? ______________________________

Case 15-13: Neonatal Cystourethrogram

LOCATION: Inpatient, Hospital

PATIENT: Crystal Morgan

ATTENDING PHYSICIAN: Rolando Ortez, MD

RADIOLOGIST: Morton Monson, MD

CLINICAL SYMPTOMS: Congenital hydronephrosis.

VOIDING URETHROCYSTOGRAPHY: The study is technically limited due to the infant's inability to cooperate. The urinary bladder was filled to presumed capacity before spontaneous voiding. The bladder capacity is estimated at 25 cc. No immediate, delayed, or voiding reflux is demonstrated.

IMPRESSION: No definite vesicoureteral reflux demonstrated.

CPT Code(s): ______________________________

ICD-10-CM Code(s): ______________________________

ICD-9-CM Code(s): ______________________________

Abstracting Questions

1. Was this an acquired or congenital condition? ______________________________
2. What type of evaluation was performed? ______________________________

Chapter 16

Interventional Radiology and Radiation Oncology

Interventional radiologists perform both the procedure and the radiologic services, so you will report both the procedure and radiology services in Chapter 16 unless directed otherwise or the report indicates some other circumstance.

Case 16-1: CT-Guided Liver Biopsy

LOCATION: Outpatient, Hospital

PATIENT: Mike Morgan

PRIMARY CARE PHYSICIAN: Ronald Green, MD

INTERVENTIONAL RADIOLOGIST: Edward Riddle, MD

EXAMINATION: CT-guided liver biopsy.

CLINICAL SYMPTOMS: Liver mass.

CT-GUIDED LIVER BIOPSY: Informed consent was obtained. The patient was placed supine on the CT table, and axial CT was performed to localize the low-density lesion within the dome of the liver medially. The right mid-axillary line skin was prepped and draped in the usual sterile fashion. The skin and subcutaneous tissues were infiltrated with 1% lidocaine. A 19-gauge coaxial needle was advanced into the low-density lesion, and axial CT was performed to confirm needle position prior to biopsy. Four 20-gauge core biopsy samples were obtained. Biopsy samples were obtained using a 20-gauge Monotype biopsy gun. The biopsy gun and coaxial needle were removed.

The patient did not receive conscious sedation. His pulse oximeter and vital signs were monitored throughout the exam. There were no complications. He tolerated the procedure well and left the radiology department in stable condition.

IMPRESSION: Successful and uncomplicated CT-guided biopsy of a low-density mass within the dome of the liver medially.

Pathology Report Later Indicated: Primary malignancy of the liver.

CPT Code(s): ______________________________

ICD-10-CM Code(s): ______________________________

ICD-9-CM Code(s): ______________________________

Abstracting Questions

1. What technique was used to accomplish the liver biopsy? ______________________________
2. What type of radiological guidance was used? ______________________________
3. Was the radiological guidance reported separately? ______________________________
4. Was sedation administered? ______________________________

Case 16-2: CT-Guided Lung Mass Biopsy

Report the services, diagnosis, and sedation (administered by Dr. Riddle) provided to this patient.

LOCATION: Outpatient, Hospital

PATIENT: Susan Potter

PRIMARY CARE PHYSICIAN: Frank Gaul, MD

INTERVENTIONAL RADIOLOGIST: Edward Riddle, MD

EXAMINATION: CT-guided right lung mass biopsy.

CLINICAL SYMPTOMS: Right lung mass.

CT-GUIDED RIGHT LUNG MASS BIOPSY: Informed consent was obtained from this 33-year-old patient. The patient was placed prone on the CT table, and axial CT was performed to localize a pulmonary nodule within the right lower lobe of the right lung. Skin over the right back was prepped and draped in the usual sterile fashion. Skin and subcutaneous tissues were infiltrated with 1% lidocaine. A 19-gauge coaxial needle was advanced into the pulmonary node in the right lower lobe. Axial CT was performed to confirm needle position prior to biopsy. Three 20-gauge core biopsy samples were obtained using a 20-gauge Monopty biopsy gun. Coaxial needle and biopsy gun were removed.

The patient received conscious sedation. Her pulse oximeter and vital signs were monitored throughout the exam. There were no complications. She tolerated the procedure well and left the radiology department in stable condition. The total time of sedation was 30 minutes.

IMPRESSION: Successful and uncomplicated CT-guided core biopsy of nodule within the lower lobe of the lung.

Pathology Report Later Indicated: Primary malignancy of the lung.

CPT Code(s): ______________________________

ICD-10-CM Code(s): ______________________________

ICD-9-CM Code(s): ______________________________

Abstracting Questions

1. Why do you report modifier -RT on the CPT code? ______________________________
2. What is a Monopty biopsy gun? ______________________________

Case 16-3: Lumbar Puncture

LOCATION: Outpatient, Hospital

PATIENT: Dori Gonzalez

PRIMARY CARE PHYSICIAN: Leslie Alanda, MD

INTERVENTIONAL RADIOLOGIST: Edward Riddle, MD

EXAMINATION: Lumbar puncture.

CLINICAL SYMPTOMS: Headache.

LUMBAR PUNCTURE: Procedure, risks, and goals of fluoroscopic-guided lumbar puncture were discussed with the patient, who verbalized an understanding and wished to proceed. Following the usual sterile prep and local anesthesia, a 20-gauge spinal needle was inserted into the subarachnoid space at L4-5. Approximately 3.5 cc of clear CSF was obtained and sent for requested tests. No immediate complications were evident.

Cytologic Pathology Report Later Indicated: No abnormality within spinal fluid.

CPT Code(s): ____________________

ICD-10-CM Code(s): ____________________

ICD-9-CM Code(s): ____________________

Abstracting Questions

1. What type of radiological guidance was utilized? ____________________
2. Was there a pathology report for the lumbar puncture? ____________________

Case 16-4: Ultrasound-Guided Paracentesis

Note that this patient received conscious sedation (administered by Dr. Riddle), which is to be reported.

LOCATION: Outpatient, Hospital

PATIENT: Kenneth Anderson

PRIMARY CARE PHYSICIAN: Ronald Green, MD

INTERVENTIONAL RADIOLOGIST: Edward Riddle, MD

EXAMINATION: Ultrasound-guided paracentesis.

CLINICAL SYMPTOMS: Cirrhosis, massive ascites, abdominal discomfort.

ULTRASOUND-GUIDED PARACENTESIS: Informed consent was obtained from this 56-year-old patient. The right abdomen was prepped and draped in the usual sterile fashion. Skin and subcutaneous tissues were infiltrated with 1% lidocaine. A 5 French Yueh catheter was placed into the fluid within the peritoneal cavity using ultrasound guidance. Sixty cubic centimeters of clear, dark yellow fluid was aspirated and sent to the lab for requested analysis. An additional 10 liters of fluid was removed for therapeutic purposes. Fluid was removed using a vacuum bottle.

The paracentesis catheter was removed. The patient received conscious sedation for 30 minutes. His pulse oximeter and vital signs were monitored throughout the exam. There were no complications. He tolerated the procedure well and left the radiology department in stable condition.

IMPRESSION: Successful and uncomplicated ultrasound-guided paracentesis. Sixty cubic centimeters of fluid was sent to the lab for analysis. A total of 10 liters of fluid was removed for therapeutic purposes.

CPT Code(s): ______________________________

ICD-10-CM Code(s): ______________________________

ICD-9-CM Code(s): ______________________________

Abstracting Questions

1. Was this an initial or subsequent paracentesis? ______________________________
2. What type of radiological guidance was utilized? ______________________________
3. What types of anesthesia were used? ______________________________

Case 16-5: Catheter Placement

Report the services, diagnosis(es), and any sedation provided to this patient by the interventional radiologist.

LOCATION: Outpatient, Hospital

PATIENT: John Cane

PRIMARY CARE PHYSICIAN: Rapheal White, MD

INTERVENTIONAL RADIOLOGIST: Edward Riddle, MD

EXAMINATION: Right IVJ Port-a-Cath placement.

CLINICAL SYMPTOMS: Primary lung cancer. Access required for chemotherapy.

PORT-A-CATH PLACEMENT: Informed consent was obtained from this 26-year-old patient. The right neck and infraclavicular region were prepped and draped in the usual sterile fashion. Skin and subcutaneous tissues were infiltrated with 1% lidocaine with epinephrine. Under ultrasound guidance, access was obtained into the right jugular vein, and over a 0.035 J-tip guidewire the needle was exchanged for a 10 French peel-away sheath. A subcutaneous pocket was created in the right infraclavicular region using blunt dissection. A 9.6 French Bard single-lumen Port-a-Cath was placed into the pocket and a subcutaneous tunnel created from the pocket to the right IJV puncture site. The 9.6 French catheter was advanced through the tunnel and placed through the peel-away sheath. The sheath was removed. Under fluoroscopic observation the distal tip of the catheter was positioned in the right atrium. The pocket was closed using subcutaneous interrupted sutures with 4–0 Vicryl and a subcuticular stitch with 4–0 Vicryl. The right neck incision site was closed using vertical mattress suture technique with 3–0 Ethilon.

Patient received conscious sedation for 45 minutes. The patient's pulse oximeter and vital signs were monitored throughout the exam. There were no complications. The patient tolerated the procedure well and left the radiology department in stable condition.

A single digital spot radiograph obtained demonstrates the single-lumen port placed via a right IJV approach with the distal tip of the catheter in the right atrium.

CPT Code(s): ______________________________

ICD-10-CM Code(s): ______________________________

ICD-9-CM Code(s): ______________________________

Abstracting Questions

1. Was the catheter inserted by the radiologist? ______________________________
2. Was the catheter inserted into the venous or arterial system? ______________________________
3. Was the catheter inserted centrally or peripherally? ______________________________
4. Was the catheter tunneled? ______________________________
5. Was a subcutaneous port/pump inserted? ______________________________
6. Does the age of the patient affect code assignment? ______________________________
7. What were the two types of guidance used? ______________________________
8. The catheter inserted was used for access for what purpose? ______________________________

Case 16-6: Carotid Angiogram

LOCATION: Outpatient, Hospital

PATIENT: Bill Yates

PRIMARY CARE PHYSICIAN: Ronald Green, MD

INTERVENTIONAL RADIOLOGIST: Edward Riddle, MD

EXAMINATION: Arch aorta with right and left carotid arteriograms and right and left cerebral arteriograms.

CLINICAL SYMPTOMS: Carotid artery stenosis.

ANGIOGRAPHIC TECHNIQUE: Informed consent was obtained. The right groin was prepped and draped in the usual sterile fashion. Skin and subcutaneous tissues were infiltrated with 1% lidocaine. Access was obtained in the right common femoral artery, and over a 0.035 Benson guidewire the needle was exchanged for a 5 French sheath. Over the guidewire a 5 French Simmons catheter was placed into the aortic arch and contrast was injected, and catheterization was performed using the brachiocephalic artery and a 0.035 angled guidewire. The left common carotid artery was selectively catheterized using the guidewire and a Simmons II catheter. Left carotid arteriogram was performed in multiple projections during mechanical injection of contrast through the catheter. AP and lateral cerebral arteriograms were also obtained during mechanical injection of contrast through the catheter.

The right carotid artery was selectively catheterized using the angled Glidewire and Simmons II catheter. Right carotid arteriogram was performed in multiple projections during mechanical injection of contrast through the catheter. AP and lateral right cerebral arteriography was also performed during mechanical injection of contrast through the catheter.

The catheter and sheath were removed. Hemostasis was obtained using a 6 French AngioSeal device. The patient received conscious sedation. His pulse oximeter and vital signs were monitored throughout the exam. There were no complications. The patient tolerated the procedure well and left the radiology department in stable condition.

ARCH AORTOGRAM: Normal variant bovine arch is present. Origins of the gray vessels are widely patent. Visualized bilateral subclavian arteries are patent, as are the bilateral vertebral arteries.

LEFT CAROTID ARTERIOGRAM: Common carotid artery is patent. There is 60-65% narrowing of the distal common carotid artery involving the bulb. The origin of the external carotid artery demonstrates 30-40% diameter narrowing as a result of the left carotid bulb narrowing. The internal carotid artery is widely patent. There is significant tortuosity of the proximal to mid internal carotid artery, with no other stenosis seen.

RIGHT CAROTID ARTERIOGRAM: Right common artery is widely patent, including the bulb. Internal and external carotid arteries are also widely patent. There is significant tortuosity of the proximal to mid internal carotid artery. No stenosis is identified.

LEFT CEREBRAL ARTERIOGRAM: The intracranial internal carotid artery is patent. Anterior middle and middle cerebral arteries are patent with no stenosis noted. No aneurysm is identified. No hypervascular or hypovascular mass is seen.

RIGHT CEREBRAL ARTERIOGRAM: Intracranial internal carotid artery demonstrates no stenosis. Anterior middle cerebral arteries are widely patent with no stenosis seen. No aneurysm is noted. No hypervascular or hypovascular mass is identified.

IMPRESSION
1. Normal variant bovine arch.
2. Negative right and left cerebral arteriograms.
3. 60-65% diameter narrowing of the distal left carotid bulb.
4. Patent bilateral internal carotid arteries with significant tortuosity of the proximal to mid cervical internal carotid arteries.

CPT Code(s): ______________________________

ICD-10-CM Code(s): ______________________________

ICD-9-CM Code(s): ______________________________

Abstracting Questions

1. What was the initial insertion site for the catheter? ______________________________
2. Was the left common carotid selective placement first or second order? ______________________________
3. Was the right carotid selective placement first, second, or third order? ______________________________
4. How many arteriogram codes were assigned? ______________________________
5. Was contrast used during the procedures? ______________________________
6. Does the use of contrast affect the code selection? ______________________________
7. Was the conscious (moderate) sedation reported? ______________________________

Case 16-7: Aortogram

LOCATION: Outpatient, Hospital

PATIENT: Theodore Lambert

PRIMARY CARE PHYSICIAN: Ronald Green, MD

INTERVENTIONAL RADIOLOGIST: Edward Riddle, MD

EXAMINATION: Arch aortogram with bilateral carotid and cerebral arteriograms.

CLINICAL SYMPTOMS: Previous stroke; carotid artery stenosis.

AORTOGRAPHIC TECHNIQUE: Informed consent was obtained. The right groin was prepped and draped in the usual sterile fashion. Skin and subcutaneous tissues were infiltrated with 1% lidocaine. Access was obtained of the right common femoral artery, and over a 0.035 Bentson guidewire the needle was exchanged for a 5 French sheath. Over the guidewire a 5 French Pigtail catheter was threaded to the aortic arch and angiography was performed in the LAO projection during mechanical injection of contrast through the catheter. The catheter was exchanged for a 5 French H1H catheter. The right vertebral artery was selectively catheterized using the H1H and a 0.035 angled Glidewire. Posterior fossa arteriogram was performed during hand injection of contrast through the catheter. This was performed in AP and lateral projections.

The right common carotid artery was selectively catheterized using the Glidewire and H1H catheter. Right carotid arteriogram was performed in three projections during mechanical injection of contrast through the catheter. AP and lateral cerebral arteriography on the right was performed during mechanical injection of contrast through the catheter.

The left common carotid artery was selectively catheterized using the Glidewire and H1H. Left carotid arteriogram was performed during hand injection of contrast through the catheter. Cerebral arteriogram was performed on the left during hand injection of contrast through the catheter.

Catheter and sheath were removed. Hemostasis was obtained using a 6 French AngioSeal device. The patient received conscious sedation. His pulse oximeter and vital signs were monitored throughout the exam. There were no complications. He tolerated the procedure well and left the radiology department in stable condition.

ARCH AORTOGRAM: The arch is unremarkable. Origins of the great vessels are normal in caliber with no stenosis seen. Subclavian arteries are patent. Bilateral vertebral arteries are patent. Left common carotid artery is small in caliber and indicates that the left internal carotid artery is completely occluded.

POSTERIOR FOSSA ARTERIOGRAM: Visualized distal right vertebral artery is patent. Basilar artery is unremarkable, as are the bilateral posterior cerebral arteries. No aneurysm is seen. No anterior cerebral arterial circulation is noted on this posterior fossa injection.

RIGHT CAROTID ARTERIOGRAM: Calcified atheromatous disease of the carotid bulb and proximal internal carotid artery is noted. There is approximately 30-40% diameter narrowing of the carotid bulb, with no significant stenosis seen involving the proximal internal carotid artery. There is a 90-95% diameter narrowing of the proximal external carotid artery.

LEFT CAROTID ARTERIOGRAM: The common carotid artery is small in caliber, with the distal common carotid artery demonstrating a high-grade stenosis with a "string sign." The internal carotid artery is completely occluded.

RIGHT CEREBRAL ARTERIOGRAM: The distal internal carotid artery and the intracranial internal carotid artery are widely patent. The right anterior and middle cerebral artery and their distribution are unremarkable, with no stenosis seen. No hypervascular or hypovascular mass is present. No aneurysm is seen. The left anterior and middle cerebral arterial supply is provided via a patent anterior communicating artery. No abnormalities are seen on the left anterior or middle cerebral arterial supply.

LEFT CEREBRAL ARTERIOGRAM: As discussed above, the left cerebral anterior circulation is provided from the right cerebral anterior circulation. There is no intracranial supply on the left seen via external carotid branches. No reconstitution of the left internal carotid artery is seen.

IMPRESSION
1. Negative arch aortogram with a small-caliber left common carotid artery.
2. Negative posterior fossa arteriogram.
3. 30-40% diameter narrowing of the carotid bulb on the right, with no significant stenosis of the right internal carotid artery seen.
4. Complete occlusion of the left internal carotid artery.
5. The left anterior and middle cerebral arteries receive their supply via patent anterior communicating artery from the right anterior arterial circulation.

CPT Code(s): ____________________

ICD-10-CM Code(s): ____________________

ICD-9-CM Code(s): ____________________

Abstracting Questions

1. What does LAO stand for? ____________________
2. In the Left Carotid Arteriogram section of the report, the radiologist refers to a "string sign." What is a string sign?

   ____

Case 16-8: Tube Placement

LOCATION: Outpatient, Hospital

PATIENT: Trent Quintan

PRIMARY CARE PHYSICIAN: Ronald Green, MD

INTERVENTIONAL RADIOLOGIST: Edward Riddle, MD

EXAMINATION: Gastrojejunostomy tube placement.

CLINICAL SYMPTOMS: Pre-existing gastrojejunostomy tube migrated from the jejunum into the patient's oropharynx; tube removed and Foley catheter put in place; access required for feedings.

GASTROJEJUNOSTOMY TUBE PLACEMENT: Informed consent was obtained. The patient was placed supine on the angiographic table. Pre-existing Foley catheter was injected with contrast to evaluate its distal tip position. Through the Foley catheter a 0.035 stiff-angled Glidewire was advanced into the jejunum. The Foley catheter was removed. An 18 French 2.3 cm MIC KEY J tube was cut and fed over the wire. The MIC KEY was secured in place. Contrast was injected into the tube to confirm catheter tip position.

There were no complications. The patient tolerated the procedure well and left the radiology department in stable condition.

FEEDING TUBE INJECTION: The new MIC KEY feeding tube distal tip is seen within the distal duodenum rather than extending into the patient's jejunum.

IMPRESSION: Successful and uncomplicated placement of a new 18 French 2.3 cm MIC KEY feeding tube.

CPT Code(s): ______________________________

ICD-10-CM Code(s): ______________________________

ICD-9-CM Code(s): ______________________________

Abstracting Questions

1. Was this an initial tube placement or a replacement? ______________________________
2. The tube had migrated to this location? ______________________________
3. Is the fluoroscopic guidance reported separately? ______________________________
4. The diagnosis is reported with a ______________________________ code.

Case 16-9: Fistulogram

LOCATION: Outpatient, Hospital

PATIENT: Myron Colter

PRIMARY CARE PHYSICIAN: Ronald Green, MD

INTERVENTIONAL RADIOLOGIST: Edward Riddle, MD

EXAMINATION: Left arm fistulogram.

CLINICAL SYMPTOMS: Native radiocephalic fistula with multiple aneurysms of fistula; questionable stenosis; renal failure.

LEFT ARM FISTULOGRAM: Informed consent was obtained. The left wrist and forearm were prepped and draped in the usual sterile fashion. The skin and subcutaneous tissues were infiltrated with 1% lidocaine. Access was obtained in the fistula near the wrist using a micropuncture needle. Over 0.018 guidewire the needle was exchanged for a 5 French micropuncture dilator. Fistulogram was performed during hand injection of contrast through the dilator. Contrast was refluxed to the arterial anastomosis. The dilator was removed. Hemostatic was obtained using manual compression to the puncture site.

There is a native radiocephalic fistula. The arterial anastomosis is widely patent. Tortuosity of the native radial artery is seen. There is no stenosis seen involving the cephalic vein in its entire length. Aneurysmal dilatation involving the vein within the left forearm is noted. Tortuosity of the vein is seen, again with no focal stenosis identified. Collateral filling of brachial veins is seen. Axillary, subclavian, and innominate veins are patent. The superior vena cava is patent.

The patient did not receive conscious sedation. His pulse oximeter and vital signs were monitored throughout the exam. There were no complications. He tolerated the procedure well and left the radiology department in stable condition.

IMPRESSION: Tortuosity of the cephalic vein involving the left forearm with aneurysmal dilatation noted to be most prominent in two focal areas. No stenosis is identified involving the native fistula. No central venous stenosis or occlusion is seen.

CPT Code(s): ______________________________

ICD-10-CM Code(s): ______________________________

ICD-9-CM Code(s): ______________________________

Abstracting Questions

1. What vessels were involved in the fistula? ______________________________
2. The catheterization would be listed in the CPT index under the main term "Catheterization" and what subterm?

   ____

Case 16-10: Extremity Angiogram

LOCATION: Outpatient, Hospital

PATIENT: George Ball

PRIMARY CARE PHYSICIAN: Ronald Green, MD

SURGEON: Gary Sanchez, MD

INTERVENTIONAL RADIOLOGIST: Edward Riddle, MD

EXAMINATION: Right lower extremity angiogram and thrombolysis.

CLINICAL SYMPTOMS: Cold right foot.

RIGHT LOWER EXTREMITY ANGIOGRAM AND THROMBOLYSIS: This 62-year-old male presented a month ago with ischemic changes below the knee of the right lower extremity. Some years earlier, the patient had a femoral-popliteal Gore-Tex graft placed. At the time of the angiogram a month ago, there was clot of virtually all the arteries commencing in the distal external iliac artery. We saw very few collateralizations extending into the right lower extremity. Subsequent lytic procedure cleared the Gore-Tex graft and the popliteal artery, but there was then very hard material in the distal popliteal artery that was resistant to the tPA lysis. Subsequently, the patient was taken to the operating room by Dr. Sanchez, where he placed a vein graft from the proximal third of the Gore-Tex graft and inserted it into the posterior tibial artery. The patient then did very well. He now presents acutely with ischemic changes of the right foot.

The patient is on heparin and had been taking Plavix and aspirin as an outpatient. The present procedure was performed via the left femoral artery with single-wall micropuncture entry and placement of a 5 French sheath. A 5 French Omni Flush catheter was then positioned into the right external iliac artery for examination of the right lower extremity.

There is a patency of the right external iliac artery to the junction with the common femoral artery. The common femoral artery is virtually occluded. One or two proximal branches are arising from the artery. The superficial femoral artery and the Gore-Tex graft are occluded. There was also no visualization of the saphenous vein graft. Some collaterals from the deep femoral artery can be visualized at the level of the knee. Although these are scant, they are certainly more than we appreciated when the patient initially arrived here last month.

Utilizing a long Glidewire, I obtained access into the Gore-Tex graft. While traversing the Gore-Text graft, I kept the curve of the wire pointed anteromedially, hoping that we might enter the vein graft. I was able to extend the Glidewire all the way to the knee. Subsequently, a Mewissen catheter with 15 cm of holes was placed proximally with the most proximal hole in the beginning of the clot in the common femoral artery. Coaxially, a Katzen wire with 12 cm of holes was positioned into the graft. tPA was then commenced through both catheters. The patient was medicated with intravenous Versed and fentanyl. He will return to the angiographic suite in the morning.

IMPRESSION: Complete occlusion of the patient's superficial femoral artery, Gore-Tex femoral-popliteal graft, and saphenous graft that extends from the Gore-Tex graft to the posterior tibial artery. Coaxial system has been appropriately placed and tPA lysis started.

CPT Code(s): ____

ICD-10-CM Code(s): ____

ICD-9-CM Code(s): ____

Abstracting Questions

1. The furthest extent of this selective catheterization was to what vessel ____________ ____________ artery and to this order? ______________________________________

Case 16-11: Abdominal Aortogram

LOCATION: Outpatient, Hospital

PATIENT: Russell Wallace

PRIMARY CARE PHYSICIAN: Ronald Green, MD

INTERVENTIONAL RADIOLOGIST: Edward Riddle, MD

EXAMINATION: CO_2 abdominal aortogram with right and left lower extremity arteriograms.

CLINICAL SYMPTOMS: Transplanted kidney; nonhealing ulcer of the left heel.

CO_2 ABDOMINAL AORTOGRAM WITH RIGHT AND LEFT LOWER EXTREMITY ARTERIOGRAMS: Informed consent was obtained from this 44-year-old patient. The right groin was prepped and draped in the usual sterile fashion. The skin and subcutaneous tissues were infiltrated with 1% lidocaine. Access was obtained into the right common femoral artery, and over a 0.035 Benson guidewire a 5 French Omni-Flush catheter was placed into the abdominal aorta. CO_2 abdominal aortogram was performed during hand injection of CO_2 through the catheter. The catheter was pulled down to above the aortic bifurcation and right, and left anterior oblique pelvic arteriography was obtained during hand injection of CO_2 through the catheter. Access was obtained in the left common femoral artery using a 0.035 angled Glidewire and Omni-Flush catheter. Left lower extremity arteriogram was performed using interactive bolus chase technique during mechanical injection of contrast through the catheter. Arterial pressures were measured from the left common femoral artery with pullback pressures obtained into the abdominal aorta. In addition, the aortic pressures were measured with pullback pressures obtained into the right common femoral artery. The catheter was removed. Right lower extremity arteriogram was obtained during mechanical injection of contrast through the sidearm of the sheath in the right groin.

The sheath was removed. Hemostasis was obtained using a 6 French AngioSeal device. The patient received conscious sedation. His pulse oximeter and vital signs were monitored throughout the exam. There were no complications. He tolerated the procedure well and left the radiology department in stable condition.

ABDOMINAL AORTOGRAM: There is no angiographic evidence for infrarenal abdominal aortic aneurysm. No hemodynamically significant stenosis of the aorta is seen. Renal arteries are not identified.

RIGHT LOWER EXTREMITY ARTERIOGRAM: Transplanted right pelvic kidney is seen arriving from the right external iliac artery. There is no stenosis of the right common iliac or external iliac arteries seen. Internally iliac artery appears patent. Right common femoral artery is also patent. Superficial femoral artery is patent. At and just below the level of the adductor hiatus there is mild-to-moderate atheromatous disease with approximately 50% diameter narrowing of the artery seen in the focal area involving the proximal popliteal artery. The remainder of the popliteal artery is patent. Anterior tibial artery occludes proximally. Tibioperoneal trunk is patent. Posterior tibial artery occludes proximally. Peroneal atheromatous changes are seen.

LEFT LOWER EXTREMITY ARTERIOGRAM: The common, internal, and external iliac arteries are patent, as is the common femoral artery. Superficial femoral artery is also patent with no stenosis seen. Popliteal artery distally is completely occluded. Multiple collateral vessels are seen with scattered collateral filling of a peroneal artery. Distally, collaterals appear to faintly fill the dorsalis pedis with poor runoff seen into the mid-to-distal foot. Posterior tibial artery is completely occluded.

IMPRESSION
1. No aortoiliac stenosis detected. No blood pressure gradient was detected from the left common femoral artery into the abdominal aorta or from the abdominal aorta into the right common femoral artery.
2. Right pelvic transplanted kidney.
3. Mild-to-moderate distal SFA/proximal popliteal artery atheromatous disease with focal 50% diameter narrowing.
4. Poor runoff of the right lower extremity below the knee with complete occlusion of the proximal anterior and posterior tibial arteries with a severely diseased peroneal artery noted.
5. Patent left SFA with complete occlusion of the distal left popliteal artery. Multiple collateral arteries are seen providing runoff to the distal leg and proximal left foot with a small-caliber but poorly filling dorsalis pedis artery noted.

Sedation lasted 45 minutes.

CPT Code(s): ____________________

ICD-10-CM Code(s): ____________________

ICD-9-CM Code(s): ____________________

Abstracting Questions

1. Was the conscious sedation reported separately? ____________________
2. The approach for this procedure was by way of what artery? ____________________

Case 16-12: Inpatient Consultation, Radiology Oncology

CONSULTATION

LOCATION: Inpatient, Hospital

PATIENT: Don Glassheim

REQUESTING PHYSICIAN: Ronald Green, MD

CONSULTING PHYSICIAN: Rapheal White, MD

CHIEF COMPLAINT: Progression of shortness of breath with respiratory stridor associated with a large mediastinal mass.

HISTORY: This patient is a 55-year-old male who presented with progressive shortness of breath over the past several weeks. An initial chest x-ray was performed that suggested a possible pulmonary infiltrate. Reportedly, this patient's pulmonary status did not improve, and therefore a CT scan of the chest was performed that demonstrated a mediastinal mass encompassing bilateral mainstem bronchi with extrinsic compression. He underwent a mediastinoscopy. A final permanent histology demonstrates a poorly differentiated small-cell lung cancer. His respiratory status has continued to deteriorate, and he required heavy sedation with intubation and mechanical ventilation.

PAST MEDICAL HISTORY: Significant for COPD, hypercholesterolemia, and dyspepsia.

CURRENT MEDICATIONS: Lipitor, inhaler, Pepcid, aspirin, dexamethasone.

SOCIAL HISTORY: The patient is married and lives independently. He does have a significant smoking history and smokes approximately one-half pack of cigarettes per day; uses alcohol infrequently.

FAMILY HISTORY: Unobtainable.

REVIEW OF SYSTEMS: Significant for progressive shortness of breath with overall respiratory deterioration as well as a 15-lb weight loss over the past several weeks. Review of systems is otherwise negative.

PHYSICAL EXAMINATION: The patient is heavily sedated at this time. Pulse 90. Respirations 18. Head: Normocephalic and atraumatic. The auricular canals and tympanic membranes are clear and intact bilaterally. Eyes: Equal, round, and reactive. Sclera is clear. Oral cavity is pink and moist without mucosal lesions. Endotracheal tube is appreciated. Neck is supple with a midline trachea without adenopathy, thyromegaly, or JVD. Lungs are tight and have rales and rhonchi with wheezing bilaterally. Heart is regular without murmur. Abdomen is soft without hepatosplenomegaly, mass, tenderness, rebound, or guarding. Back and Extremities: No evidence of cyanosis, clubbing, edema, or focal reproducible tenderness. Neurologic: Patient again heavily sedated. Skin: No rash or lesions; has excellent turgor.

SIGNIFICANT DATA: CT scan and chest x-ray have been reviewed and visualized with the results as outlined.

IMPRESSION: Poorly differentiated small-cell lung cancer with full staging not performed at this time but associated with a significant respiratory deterioration.

RECOMMENDATIONS: This is a 55-year-old male with small-cell lung cancer associated with bilateral extrinsic compression on both mainstem bronchi. We do believe local radiotherapy to the mediastinum may improve his respiratory status and may be performed while he is sedated and on a ventilator. We have discussed with the family regarding the indication, goals, and side effects of external beam radiotherapy. We would recommend 12 Gy in three fractions to his mediastinum. After delivery of his external beam radiotherapy, we would reassess his pulmonary status to determine if he may proceed with more standardized radiotherapy technique using concurrent chemotherapy. The family appears to understand and have vocalized their desire to proceed with this option. Therefore, the patient will undergo a simulation and treatment planning, with initiation of his radiotherapy thereafter. We appreciate the opportunity to advise you in the care of your patient.

CPT Code(s): ______________________________

ICD-10-CM Code(s): ______________________________

ICD-9-CM Code(s): ______________________________

Abstracting Questions

1. What section of CPT code was referenced to report this service? ______________________________

Case 16-13: Treatment Planning Note, Radiation Oncology

TREATMENT PLANNING NOTE

LOCATION: Inpatient, Hospital

PATIENT: Don Glassheim

ATTENDING PHYSICIAN: Ronald Green, MD

ONCOLOGIST: Rapheal White, MD

DIAGNOSIS: Poorly differentiated small-cell lung cancer with bilateral extrinsic compression of both mainstem bronchi associated with significant respiratory distress and stridor requiring heavy sedation and mechanical ventilation.

CLINICAL CONSIDERATIONS: This 55-year-old patient has small-cell lung cancer with significant respiratory distress requiring sedation and intubation with mechanical ventilation. We believe local radiotherapy may improve his respiratory status.

Medication, goals, and side effects of local radiotherapy have been discussed in detail. Since the patient is heavily sedated, his family has granted permission to proceed with this option.

TECHNICAL CONSIDERATIONS: The initial target volume will include the mediastinum, to be treated for a total of three fractions using a hypofractionation technique.

The prescribed dose would be 12 Gy in 3 fractions to the mediastinum using an AP-PA technique at 100 SAD.

The radiotherapy treatment will require a simple simulation and dose calculations. Following the simulation the patient will proceed with his mediastinal radiation. All questions have been addressed.

CPT Code(s): ______________________________

ICD-10-CM Code(s): ______________________________

ICD-9-CM Code(s): ______________________________

Abstracting Questions

1. Was the planning simple, intermediate, or complex? ______________________________

Case 16-14: Simulation Note, Radiation Oncology

SIMULATION NOTE

LOCATION: Inpatient, Hospital

PATIENT: Don Glassheim

ATTENDING PHYSICIAN: Ronald Green, MD

ONCOLOGIST: Rapheal White, MD

DIAGNOSIS: Poorly differential small-cell lung cancer with bilateral extrinsic compression on both mainstem bronchi that has required heavy sedation and intubation with mechanical ventilation. His family has elected to proceed with local radiotherapy in hopes of improving his respiratory status.

SIMULATION: After explaining simulation to the patient's family, the patient was placed on the treatment table in the supine position. The treatment volume was clinically set at 100 SAD. The initial treatment field was measured at 10 × 10 cm. The port film confirmed that the field needed to be shifted 1 cm to the left, and the field was enlarged to 12 × 12 cm. A second simulation film confirmed that the desired setup had been obtained.

Dose calculations will be performed to ensure that the prescribed dose will be delivered to the treatment volume. No blocks will be used for this course of treatment.

The entire simulation took approximately 30 minutes. The patient tolerated the procedure fairly well and will receive his first of three radiation treatments very shortly.

CPT Code(s): ____________________

ICD-10-CM Code(s): ____________________

ICD-9-CM Code(s): ____________________

Abstracting Questions

1. Was the simulation simple, intermediate, complex, or 3-D? ____________________
2. Was the enlargement of the field reported as an additional simulation? ____________________

Chapter 17
Urology

Make sure to check evolve learning system for the latest content updates

Case 17-1: Native Kidney Biopsy

Dr. Monson, radiologist, provided the ultrasound guidance service for the following procedure. Code only Dr. Avila's services.

OPERATIVE REPORT

LOCATION: Outpatient, Hospital

PATIENT: Corrine Longworth

PHYSICIAN: Ira Avila, MD

PROCEDURE PERFORMED: Native kidney biopsy.

INDICATIONS: Hematuria.

PROCEDURE: After obtaining consent and looking at the left kidney with ultrasound, the area was prepped in the usual fashion while the patient was in the prone position. For local anesthesia, 1% lidocaine was used. Multiple core biopsies were obtained without difficulty from the left kidney under real-time ultrasound guidance. Tissue was sent for light and electron microscopy and immunofluorescence.

The patient tolerated the procedure well without immediate complications. She was sent back to the outpatient procedure area. Hemoglobin will be done in 6 hours. She should be on bed rest.

Pathology Report Later Indicated: Negative for any abnormalities.

CPT Code(s): ______________________________

ICD-10-CM Code(s): ______________________________

ICD-9-CM Code(s): ______________________________

Abstracting Questions

1. What was the approach utilized for this biopsy? ______________________________
2. What does the term "native" kidney mean? ______________________________

Case 17-2: Cystoscopy

OPERATIVE REPORT

LOCATION: Outpatient, Hospital

PATIENT: Paul Oberbright

PHYSICIAN: Ira Avila, MD

PREOPERATIVE DIAGNOSIS: Prior transitional cell carcinoma of the bladder.

POSTOPERATIVE DIAGNOSIS: Recurrent transitional cell carcinoma of the bladder.

PROCEDURE PERFORMED: Cystoscopy.

CLINICAL NOTE: The patient had a superficial bladder tumor resected from around his left ureteric orifices earlier this year. He has been asymptomatic and recurrence-free since then. He missed his appointment for IVP today, so we have not visualized his upper tracts.

PROCEDURE: The patient was prepped and draped in the supine position. The urethra was anesthetized with 2% Xylocaine jelly and the patient cystoscoped. The urethra was normal. The prostate was small and nonobstructive. Inspection of the bladder demonstrated two small superficial recurrences on the right superior lateral wall. The previous resection site was clear.

ASSESSMENT: The patient will be scheduled for cystoscopy, bladder tumor resection, and retrograde pyelography in the very near future. I have already talked to him about the rationale for BCG, options, expected outcome, and complications. We will probably proceed then with BCG therapy following this.

CPT Code(s): ______________________________

ICD-10-CM Code(s): ______________________________

ICD-9-CM Code(s): ______________________________

Abstracting Questions

1. Was this procedure diagnostic or therapeutic? ______________________________
2. During the procedure, what was identified in the bladder? ______________________________

Case 17-3: Catheterization

INTRAOPERATIVE CONSULTATION AND OPERATIVE REPORT

LOCATION: Inpatient, Hospital

PATIENT: Allen Adnitha

ATTENDING PHYSICIAN: Ronald Green, MD

CONSULTANT: Ira Avila, MD

PROCEDURE PERFORMED: Catheterization.

CLINICAL INDICATIONS/NOTE: The patient is an 84-year-old gentleman who had recently undergone craniotomy. He was confused and pulled out his catheter, and nursing staff was unable to reinsert.

PROCEDURE: The patient was prepped and draped in the supine position. Urethra was anesthetized with 2% Xylocaine jelly. A 16 French Foley catheter was inserted without difficulty to straight drainage; urine returns were clear. There was some para-Foley bleeding.

The patient probably has sustained a mild urethral injury. The catheter should be left in for at least 5 days. This will depend, of course, on how the patient does neurologically. If he does well and after 5 to 7 days could be without his Foley catheter, this could be removed at that time.

CPT Code(s): ______________________________

ICD-10-CM Code(s): ______________________________

ICD-9-CM Code(s): ______________________________

Abstracting Questions

1. What type of catheter was placed during the procedure? ______________________________
2. Was the catheter permanent or temporary? ______________________________
3. What type of diagnosis code is reported for the difficulty with the catheter? ______________________________

Case 17-4: Cystoscopy and Retrograde Pyelogram

OPERATIVE REPORT

LOCATION: Outpatient, Hospital

PATIENT: John Bradshaw

PRIMARY CARE PHYSICIAN: Ronald Green, MD

SURGEON: Ira Avila, MD

PREOPERATIVE DIAGNOSIS: Bilateral hydronephrosis.

POSTOPERATIVE DIAGNOSES
1. No evidence of significant upper urinary tract pathology.
2. Gross prostatic hyperplasia.

PROCEDURE PERFORMED: Cystoscopy and retrograde pyelogram.

CLINICAL NOTE: This gentleman has worsening hydronephrosis and renal insufficiency. He was referred by Dr. Green. He did not have much of a postvoid residual on bladder scan. He has minimal lower urinary tract symptoms.

PROCEDURE: The patient was prepped and draped in the supine position. The urethra was anesthetized with 2% Xylocaine. Gently, the patient was cystoscoped using a flexible instrument. The prostate shows gross trilobar enlargement with a 4.5-cm prostatic urethral length and a 1- to 2-cm medial lobe. Bladder showed mild-to-moderate trabeculation. Ureteric orifices were very difficult to visualize. Bilateral retrograde pyelograms were performed and showed normal outflow collecting systems. There was no evidence of filling defects or calculi. There was no evidence of significant hydronephrosis. The system was drained well.

The patient tolerated the procedure well. He was given preoperative ampicillin and gentamicin. He will be discharged with ciprofloxacin 250 mg b.i.d. The patient was started on Flomax and thinks this may be helping somewhat with his voiding pattern, although really he has minimal symptoms. We will see him for follow-up in our clinic in 1 month for uroflow and bladder scan. We may need to proceed to TURP if he develops significant outflow obstruction.

CPT Code(s): ____________________

ICD-10-CM Code(s): ____________________

ICD-9-CM Code(s): ____________________

Abstracting Questions

1. Was the pyelogram separately reported? ____________________
2. What determines the ICD-10-CM fourth character and ICD-9-CM fifth digit for the diagnosis? ____________________
3. What does TURP mean? ____________________

Case 17-5: Kidney Biopsy

OPERATIVE REPORT

LOCATION: Outpatient, Hospital

PATIENT: Scott Waldren

PHYSICIAN: Ira Avila, MD

PROCEDURE PERFORMED: Kidney biopsy.

INDICATIONS: Gross hematuria and acute renal failure.

PROCEDURE: After obtaining consent, the patient was put in the prone position. His right kidney was localized using ultrasound. The area of the right kidney was sterilely prepped in the usual fashion. One-percent lidocaine was used for local anesthesia. The right kidney was accessed multiple times. Six core biopsies were obtained under real-time ultrasound guidance without difficulty. The patient tolerated the procedure well. Postbiopsy ultrasound showed no evidence of hematoma. The patient was sent back to the floor with 6 hours' bed rest and repeat hemoglobin in 6 hours.

Core biopsies were sent for light and electron microscopy and immunofluorescence.

CPT Code(s): ______________________________

ICD-10-CM Code(s): ______________________________

ICD-9-CM Code(s): ______________________________

Abstracting Questions

1. How many core biopsies were obtained? ______________________________
2. What type of ultrasound guidance was utilized? ______________________________

Case 17-6: Native Kidney Biopsy

Dr. Monson, radiologist, provided the ultrasound guidance service for the following procedure. Code only Dr. Avila's services.

OPERATIVE REPORT

LOCATION: Outpatient, Hospital

PATIENT: Lucy Smith

PHYSICIAN: Ira Avila, MD

PROCEDURE: Native kidney biopsy.

INDICATIONS: Nephrotic syndrome.

PROCEDURE: After obtaining consent, the patient was put in the prone position. The left kidney was seen using ultrasound. The area was prepped in the usual fashion. For local anesthesia, 1% lidocaine was used. Multiple core biopsies were obtained under real-time ultrasound guidance from the left kidney without difficulty. The patient tolerated the procedure very well without immediate complication. She was sent back to the outpatient procedure area. Hemoglobin will be obtained in 6 hours, and she will be on bed rest for 6 hours.

Pathology Report Later Indicated: Nephrotic syndrome.

CPT Code(s): ______________________________

ICD-10-CM Code(s): ______________________________

ICD-9-CM Code(s): ______________________________

Abstracting Questions

1. What is nephritic syndrome? ______________________________

Case 17-7: Ureteral Stent Change

Although this is a short report, it is challenging. There are two service codes, two Z codes/V codes, one external cause/E code, and three diagnosis codes in addition to three procedure codes. There are modifiers used to report these services. Careful reading of the notes associated with the service codes will reveal the use of these modifiers. Assign an external cause/E code to indicate how the injury occurred.

OPERATIVE REPORT

LOCATION: Outpatient, Hospital

PATIENT: Melissa Cathy Dugeon

ATTENDING PHYSICIAN: Ira Avila, MD

SURGEON: Ira Avila, MD

PREOPERATIVE DIAGNOSIS: Right ureteral stricture.

POSTOPERATIVE DIAGNOSIS: Same.

PROCEDURE PERFORMED: Cystoscopy, right ureteral stent change. Bimanual examination under anesthesia.

ANESTHESIA: IV sedation.

CLINICAL NOTE: This lady has a right ureteral stricture secondary to prior treatment for uterine sarcoma. CT scan performed a few months ago showed some straining in the right hemipelvis, although examination at that time failed to demonstrate anything that would be consistent with recurrent tumor. She is scheduled for follow-up CT scan in this regard in 1 week.

The patient tells me she has had some nocturia and urgency incontinence recently. There has been no dysuria or hematuria.

PROCEDURE: The patient was placed in the lithotomy position after IV sedation. She was prepped and draped in the lithotomy position. The 21 French cystoscope was passed into the bladder, and urine collected for culture. Inspection of the bladder demonstrated findings consistent with radiation cystitis, which was previously diagnosed. There is no frank neoplasia. The right ureteral stent was grasped and removed through the urethral meatus, and under fluoroscopic control the guidewire was advanced up the stent and the stent exchanged for a 7 French 26-cm stent in the usual fashion.

The patient tolerated the procedure well. She will be discharged with ciprofloxacin. We will also start Detrol LA 4 mg nightly to see if this helps; a renewal prescription for the next year has been given. Stent change will be arranged in 3 months. (Patient was sent home on ciprofloxacin.)

CPT Code(s): ____________________

ICD-10-CM Code(s): ____________________

ICD-9-CM Code(s): ____________________

Abstracting Questions

1. Are the removal and insertion each reported separately? ______________________
2. What type of code was assigned to report the removal of the stent? ______________________
3. Why does the patient have the stent? ______________________
4. The problem with the stent was reported as a ______________________.
5. Why did the patient initially require a stent? ______________________
6. What complication developed from the treatment? ______________________
7. What category of code was assigned to report the radiation? ______________________

Case 17-8: Multiple Bladder Biopsies

OPERATIVE REPORT

LOCATION: Outpatient, Hospital

PATIENT: Bill Cobbler

ATTENDING PHYSICIAN: Ira Avila, MD

SURGEON: Ira Avila, MD

PREOPERATIVE DIAGNOSIS: Recurrent transitional cell carcinoma plus BCG cystitis.

POSTOPERATIVE DIAGNOSES
1. Recurrent transitional cell carcinoma.
2. Recurrent transitional cell carcinoma plus BCG cystitis.

PROCEDURES PERFORMED
1. Cystoscopy.
2. Transurethral resection of recurrent bladder tumor.
3. Multiple bladder biopsies.

ANESTHESIA: General.

CLINICAL NOTE: This gentleman has had recurrent TCC, has not responded to BCG treatment, and has now undergone BCG with interferon and presents for follow-up. He is asymptomatic.

PROCEDURE: The patient was given a general endotracheal anesthetic, then prepped and draped in the lithotomy position. A 21 French cystoscope was passed into the bladder under direct vision. Inspection of the bladder demonstrated numerous hyperemic areas consistent with BCG cystitis and possible CIS. There was also a papillary recurrence in the right floor of the bladder just above and lateral to the right ureteric orifice. The areas in question were resected and the areas fulgurated until 10 cm^2 of bladder were resected. Specimens were sent for pathologic identification. An 18 French Foley catheter was inserted into the bladder and placed to straight drainage.

The patient tolerated the procedure well and was transferred to the recovery room in good condition. If pathology is positive, we will have to give careful consideration to alternative treatment for this patient. He has now not responded to BCG and interferon therapy. Mitomycin-C is an option, although the efficacy is really no greater than with the other therapies. A cystectomy might need to be considered in this patient.

Pathology Report Later Indicated: Primary, malignant bladder neoplasm.

CPT Code(s): ______________________________

ICD-10-CM Code(s): ______________________________

ICD-9-CM Code(s): ______________________________

Abstracting Questions

1. Was this procedure performed as an open procedure? ______________________
2. Does the size of bladder tumor resected affect the CPT code assignment? ______________________
3. Was recurrent primary cancer reported as the primary diagnosis? ______________________

Case 17-9: Fulguration and Penile Lesion Biopsy

LOCATION: Outpatient, Hospital

PATIENT: Bob Lawford

ATTENDING PHYSICIAN: Ira Avila, MD

SURGEON: Ira Avila, MD

PREOPERATIVE DIAGNOSES
1. Probable left renal calculus.
2. Multiple penile lesions consistent with condyloma acuminata.

POSTOPERATIVE DIAGNOSES
1. Bilateral ureteropelvic junction 1-cm left renal calculus.
2. Multiple penile lesions.

PROCEDURES PERFORMED
1. Cystoscope with bilateral retrograde pyelograms.
2. Circumcision.
3. Extensive fulguration of multiple penile lesions.

ANESTHESIA: General.

PROCEDURE: This gentleman was given a general endotracheal anesthetic, then prepped and draped in the lithotomy position. A flexible cystoscope was passed per urethra under direct vision. Urethra was normal. Prostate was not obstructed. Bladder mucosa was normal. Bilateral retrograde pyelograms were performed using a 5 French whistle-tip catheter under fluoroscopic control. Hard-copy images were obtained.

Images revealed what appeared to be bilateral ureteropelvic junction obstruction. A 1 cm stone was identified within the collecting system of the left kidney. Drainage films showed incomplete emptying after 20 minutes. The patient was not stented at this point in preference of performing diuretic renogram to document degree of obstruction bilaterally.

Circumcision was then performed using sleeve technique. The incision was extended dorsally to include a very large lesion dorsally. Hemostasis was achieved using electrocautery and chromic catgut ties. Prepuce was then reanastomosed to penile skin using 3–0 and 4–0 chromic catgut. There were numerous lesions in the glans that were fulgurated, resected, and sent for separate identification pathologically. The patient tolerated the procedure well and was transferred to recovery room.

Pathology Report Later Indicated: Condylomata acuminata.

CPT Code(s): ______________________________

ICD-10-CM Code(s): ______________________________

ICD-9-CM Code(s): ______________________________

Abstracting Questions

1. Does the method of circumcision affect code assignment? ______________________
2. What was performed via the scope? ______________________
3. Was the stone in the left kidney removed during this procedure? ______________________
4. Was the ureteropelvic obstruction only on the side with the kidney stone? ______________________

Case 17-10: Hydrocele Repair

OPERATIVE REPORT

LOCATION: Outpatient, Hospital

PATIENT: Jerry Fulcrum

ATTENDING PHYSICIAN: Ira Avila, MD

SURGEON: Ira Avila, MD

PREOPERATIVE DIAGNOSIS: Hypospadias with chordee and right hydrocele.

POSTOPERATIVE DIAGNOSIS: Hypospadias with congenital chordee and right hydrocele.

PROCEDURE PERFORMED: Right hydrocele repair and one-stage repair of hypospadias with preputial onlay flap.

ANESTHESIA: General.

CLINICAL NOTE: This 12-month-old male has a midshaft hypospadias with a very mild degree of chordee. He also has a persistent right hydrocele.

PROCEDURE: The patient was given a caudal block as well as a general mask anesthetic. He was prepped and draped in the supine position. A right inguinal incision was made. The testicular cord was identified at the level of the external ring and delivered. The gubernacular fibers were divided with electrocautery. The hydrocele sac was opened, and the partial end of it was resected and then bottled behind the testicle using 5–0 chromic. There was no evidence of communication of the hernia. The testis was then returned to the scrotum. The subcutaneous tissue was closed with 5–0 chromic and the skin with 5–0 subcuticular plain. Steri-Strip was applied.

The hypospadias was then dealt with. The patient was catheterized using an 8 French feeding tube. The first step following this was to mobilize the hooded foreskin. This was isolated on its own pedicle. Then the urethral meatus was circumscribed using the Beaver blade. Once the penile shaft skin had been mobilized, there was very minimal chordee. I did not believe it was necessary to remove the dorsal urethral plate from the region of the coronal sulcus. Saline erection was performed that showed a good straight penis without evidence of significant chordee.

The glans was incised and mobilized. The flap was then prepared and sutured to the dorsal urethra with 6–0 PDS. A mucosa-running stitch was used, and an interrupted second layer also was utilized. The glans was then further mobilized, rotated around behind and over the urethra, and secured with 5–0 Vicryl sutures. The prepuce was reanastomosed to the penile skin and the midline defect in the shaft skin closed with Vicryl suture. I had a good cosmetic appearance at the end of the procedure. The 8 French catheter was not tight on the anastomosis. It could be introduced without difficulty. A Prolene stitch was placed through the glans, and the 8 French feeding tube was cut and secured as a stent. Vaseline and Coban dressing were applied to the penis.

The patient tolerated the procedure well and was transferred to the recovery room in good condition.

CPT Code(s): ____________________

ICD-10-CM Code(s): ____________________

ICD-9-CM Code(s): ____________________

Abstracting Questions

1. Does the stage of the repair affect the code assignment? ____________________
2. Does the type of flap repair affect the code assignment? ____________________
3. Was the hydrocele excised or repaired? ____________________
4. Were any of the diagnosis codes affected by the gender of the patient? ____________________
5. Was the chordee diagnosis code for an acquired or congenital condition? ____________________

Chapter 18
General Surgery

Make sure to check evolve learning system for the latest content updates

Case 18-1: Perforated Appendicitis

LOCATION: Inpatient, Hospital

PATIENT: Laurence Hooper

ATTENDING PHYSICIAN: Gary Sanchez, MD

SURGEON: Gary Sanchez, MD

PREOPERATIVE DIAGNOSIS: Perforated appendicitis.

POSTOPERATIVE DIAGNOSIS: Perforated appendicitis.

ANESTHESIA: General.

PROCEDURE: The patient was brought to the operating room, placed under general anesthesia, and prepped and draped sterilely. A right lower quadrant skin incision was made with a #10 blade, and dissection was carried down through the subcutaneous tissue using electrocautery. The anterior sheath of the rectus fascia was opened. The rectus was retracted medially. The posterior sheath and peritoneum were grasped with curved clamps, sharply incised, thus allowing entry into the peritoneal cavity. There were a few adhesions, which we took down sharply. We then delivered the appendix up and into the wound. We took down the mesoappendix between Kelly clamps and tied the vascular pedicles with 2–0 silk free ties. The base of the appendix was then crushed. It was tied with a 0 Vicryl. It was inverted into the base of the cecum with a 3–0 silk pursestring suture. The abdomen was then irrigated with saline until returns were clear. We closed the posterior sheath and peritoneum with running 0 Vicryl, closed the anterior sheath with interrupted 0 Vicryl, and the skin with subcuticular 4–0 undyed Vicryl. Steri-Strips and sterile Band-Aids were applied.

All sponge and needle counts were correct. Prior to leaving the operating room, the wound was anesthetized with a total of 30 cc of 0.50% Sensorcaine with epinephrine solution.

CPT Code(s): ____________________

ICD-10-CM Code(s): ____________________

ICD-9-CM Code(s): ____________________

Abstracting Questions

1. Was the approach for this procedure open or percutaneous? ______________________
2. Was the appendix ruptured? ______________________
3. Does the rupture affect the assignment of the CPT, diagnosis codes, or all types of codes? ______________________

Case 18-2: Right Inguinal Herniorrhaphy

LOCATION: Outpatient, Hospital

PATIENT: Gary Holter

ATTENDING PHYSICIAN: Gary Sanchez, MD

SURGEON: Gary Sanchez, MD

PREOPERATIVE DIAGNOSIS: Right inguinal hernia.

POSTOPERATIVE DIAGNOSIS: Right inguinal hernia.

PROCEDURE PERFORMED: Right inguinal herniorrhaphy.

ANESTHESIA: General.

PROCEDURE: This 45-year-old patient was brought to the operating room, placed under general anesthesia, and prepped and draped sterilely. A right groin skin incision was made with a #10 blade. Dissection was carried down through the subcutaneous tissues using electrocautery. The external oblique was identified and opened along the length of its fibers along the external ring. Spermatic cord was identified and looped with a Penrose drain. Hernia sac was dissected free. High ligation was then performed with a 3–0 Vicryl suture ligature and a 2–0 silk free tie. The patulous internal ring was then closed with a simple interrupted 3–0 Vicryl suture. The floor of the canal looked quite good. We then closed the external oblique with a running 3–0 Vicryl, closed Scarpa's with interrupted 3–0 Vicryl, and closed the skin with subcuticular 4–0 undyed Vicryl. Steri-Strips and sterile Band-Aids were applied.

All sponge and needle counts were correct. The patient tolerated the procedure well and was taken to the recovery room in stable condition.

CPT Code(s): ____________________

ICD-10-CM Code(s): ____________________

ICD-9-CM Code(s): ____________________

Abstracting Questions

1. What was the location of the hernia repair? ____________________
2. Define the inguinal area of the body. ____________________
3. Does the age of the patient affect code assignment? ____________________
4. Was the hernia reducible? ____________________
5. Was the procedure performed unilateral or bilateral? ____________________

Case 18-3: Laparoscopic Cholecystectomy

LOCATION: Outpatient, Hospital

PATIENT: Mable Moore

ATTENDING PHYSICIAN: Gary Sanchez, MD

SURGEON: Gary Sanchez, MD

PREOPERATIVE DIAGNOSIS: Symptomatic cholelithiasis.

POSTOPERATIVE DIAGNOSIS: Same as Preoperative.

PROCEDURE PERFORMED: Laparoscopic cholecystectomy.

ANESTHESIA: General.

PROCEDURE: The patient was brought to the operating room, placed under general anesthesia, and prepped and draped sterilely after a Foley catheter and oral gastric tubes were inserted. Supraumbilical skin incision was made with a #11 blade, and dissection was carried down through subcutaneous tissues bluntly. Midline fascia was grasped with Kocher clamp. A 0 Vicryl suture was then placed on either side of the midline fascia. A Veress needle was inserted into the abdominal cavity. A drop test confirmed placement within the peritoneal space. The abdomen was then insufflated with carbon dioxide. A 10-mm trocar port and laparoscope were introduced, showing no damage to the overlaying viscera. Under direct vision, three additional trocar ports were placed, one upper midline 10 mm and two right upper quadrant 5 mm. The gallbladder was grasped and was elevated from its fossa. The cystic duct and artery were dissected free, doubly clipped proximally and distally before dividing them with the hook scissors. The gallbladder was then shelled from its fossa using electrocautery and brought up and out of the upper midline incision. The abdomen was irrigated with saline until returns were clear. Trocar ports were then removed under direct vision with no evidence of bleeding. Supraumbilical port site fascial defect was closed with a single interrupted 0 Vicryl suture. The skin at all port sites was closed with subcuticular 4–0 undyed Vicryl. Steri-Strips and sterile Band-Aids were applied.

All sponge and needle counts were correct. The patient tolerated the procedure well and was taken to recovery in stable condition.

CPT Code(s): ______________________________

ICD-10-CM Code(s): ______________________________

ICD-9-CM Code(s): ______________________________

Abstracting Questions

1. Were there any other reportable services in addition to the removal of gallbladder? ______________
2. What was incidentally repaired during the procedure? ______________________

Case 18-4: Stab Wound

Assign an external cause code/E code to indicate how the injury occurred.

LOCATION: Inpatient, Hospital

PATIENT: Tara Barron

ATTENDING PHYSICIAN: Gary Sanchez, MD

SURGEON: Gary Sanchez, MD

PREOPERATIVE DIAGNOSIS: Stab wound, right upper quadrant.

POSTOPERATIVE DIAGNOSIS: Same as Preoperative.

PROCEDURE PERFORMED: Exploration of stab wound, right upper quadrant, with closure of fascial defect.

ANESTHESIA: General.

PROCEDURE: The patient was brought to the operating room and placed under general anesthesia; we then removed the jar lid from around the knife and the patient's clothing and prepped with Betadine solution. We extended the incision on either side of the right upper quadrant stab wound 2-3 cm and carried the dissection through subcutaneous tissues using electrocautery. We followed the knife down along its tract and then could see the knife had penetrated the anterior sheath and the rectus fascia by about a quarter inch. We removed the knife and could see the tip was just within the rectus muscle. There was no peritoneal penetration. We then closed the fascia with interrupted 0 Vicryl and closed the skin with vertical mattress 3–0 Ethilon sutures.

All sponge and needle counts were correct. Patient tolerated this well and was taken to recovery in stable condition.

CPT Code(s): ______________________________

ICD-10-CM Code(s): ______________________________

ICD-9-CM Code(s): ______________________________

Abstracting Questions

1. What is the main term in the CPT referenced for this procedure? ______________________________
2. What is the secondary term in the CPT referenced to report this procedure? ______________________________
3. Can the repair be reported separately? ______________________________
4. How far had the knife penetrated? ______________________________

Case 18-5: Left Breast Biopsy

LOCATION: Outpatient, Hospital

PATIENT: Adrienne Gardener

ATTENDING PHYSICIAN: Gary Sanchez, MD

SURGEON: Gary Sanchez, MD

PREOPERATIVE DIAGNOSIS: Left breast mass.

POSTOPERATIVE DIAGNOSIS: Left breast mass.

PROCEDURE PERFORMED: Left breast biopsy.

ANESTHESIA: Local with IV sedation.

PROCEDURE: The patient was brought to the operating room, given IV sedation, and then anesthetized with a total of 30 cc of 1% Sensorcaine with epinephrine solution. An incision was made over the top of the mass with a #15 blade, and dissection was carried down through subcutaneous tissues sharply. We encountered the mass, which appeared to be a fibroadenoma. We excised this sharply. We got the entire lesion. We controlled bleeding with electrocautery. We then closed the skin with subcuticular 4–0 undyed Vicryl. Steri-Strips and sterile Band-Aids were applied.

Patient tolerated the procedure well and was taken to the recovery room in stable condition.

Pathology Report Later Indicated: Fibroadenoma.

CPT Code(s): ______________________________

ICD-10-CM Code(s): ______________________________

ICD-9-CM Code(s): ______________________________

Abstracting Questions

1. What was the approach? ______________________________
2. Was this incisional or excisional? ______________________________
3. Does the final diagnosis affect the CPT code assignment? ______________________________

Case 18-6: Amputation

LOCATION: Inpatient, Hospital

PATIENT: Lee Laetrile

ATTENDING PHYSICIAN: Gary Sanchez, MD

SURGEON: Gary Sanchez, MD

PREOPERATIVE DIAGNOSIS: Necrotic left foot, gangrenous.

POSTOPERATIVE DIAGNOSIS: Same as Preoperative.

PROCEDURE PERFORMED: Left above-knee amputation.

ANESTHESIA: General.

PROCEDURE: The patient was brought to the operating theater and placed in the supine position on the operating room table. After receiving a spinal anesthetic, he was prepped and draped in a sterile fashion. A fish-mouth incision was marked out on the left leg. This was above the knee. Incisions were made. He has a fair amount of varicosities. These were rather ropey, large varicosities on his thigh. Most of these were on the medial aspect. These were ligated after they were transected. They were ligated either by clamps and then 3–0 Vicryl ties or 3–0 Vicryl stick ties. There was some blood loss with this. He had a very edematous leg. There was also a lot of edema in the leg, which, of course, came out of the tissues. Sharp dissection was carried down through the subcutaneous tissues all the way through the fascia and through the muscles. It came down onto the femur. This was cleared off. We used a right-angle clamp to get around the superficial femoral artery and vein. These were clamped with Lahey right angles, transected, and then ligated with 2–0 Vicryl. Proximally it was double ligated with a 2–0 Vicryl free tie and then a 2–0 silk stick tie. A periosteal elevator was used on the femur. This was taken back to about 10 cm from the proximal condyles.

I wanted to be sure that we had made our incision such that we would be a little bit more proximal than typical. Patient has had a minor problem healing his right leg, but this has basically held up. The left leg also is a concern for being able to heal, and so I wanted to be sure we were proximal enough so we could get this to heal up. The femur was transected with a Gigli saw. I then used a guillotine knife to transect the posterior muscle group. Clamps were applied to the bleeding vessels. This included the popliteal artery, which had already been transected and ligated. The sciatic nerve was infiltrated with 0.5% Marcaine with epinephrine. I then retracted and clamped it proximally and transected and ligated it with 2–0 Vicryl. Bleeding points in the muscles were oversewn with 3–0 Vicryl stick ties. The end of the bone was smoothed with a bone rasp. The wound was then irrigated out with 3 liters of kanamycin/Bacitracin in LF. The Ortholav was used for this. Surgicel was then applied into the open end of the femur in the bone marrow cavity. A 10-mm flat Jackson-Pratt drain was also placed and brought out through a separate stab wound laterally. We then closed the fascia and the muscles together using interrupted sutures of 2–0 Vicryl. The skin was then brought together with staples. Xeroform, Fluffs, Kerlix, and an Ace wrap were then applied.

The patient tolerated the procedure well and was taken to the recovery room in stable condition. I met with the patient's family postoperatively to discuss the operative findings.

CPT Code(s): ____________________

ICD-10-CM Code(s): ____________________

ICD-9-CM Code(s): ____________________

Abstracting Questions

1. What body extremity was amputated? ____________________
2. What was the level of amputation? ____________________

Case 18-7: Umbilical Herniorrhaphy

LOCATION: Outpatient, Hospital

PATIENT: Ben Bolten

ATTENDING PHYSICIAN: Gary Sanchez, MD

SURGEON: Gary Sanchez, MD

PREOPERATIVE DIAGNOSIS: Umbilical hernia.

POSTOPERATIVE DIAGNOSIS: Umbilical hernia.

PROCEDURE PERFORMED: Umbilical herniorrhaphy.

ANESTHESIA: General.

PROCEDURE: This 53-year-old patient was brought to the operating room and placed under general anesthesia, then prepped and draped sterilely. An infraumbilical skin incision was made with a #15 blade. Dissection was carried down through subcutaneous tissues using electrocautery. The hernia sac was dissected free from the umbilicus and reduced. The fascial defect was then closed with interrupted 0 Vicryl sutures. The umbilicus was tacked back down to the fascia with a 3–0 undyed Vicryl and skin closed with subcuticular 4–0 undyed Vicryl. Steri-Strips and sterile bandage were applied. All sponge and needle counts were correct. Before the patient left the operating room, the wound was anesthetized with a total of 30 cc of 0.5% Sensorcaine with epinephrine solution.

CPT Code(s): ________________________________

ICD-10-CM Code(s): ________________________________

ICD-9-CM Code(s): ________________________________

Abstracting Questions

1. Was general anesthesia utilized during this procedure? ________________________________
2. What is an infraumbilical skin incision? ________________________________

Case 18-8: Colostomy and Cholecystectomy

LOCATION: Inpatient, Hospital

PATIENT: Simon Sulten

ATTENDING PHYSICIAN: Gary Sanchez, MD

SURGEON: Gary Sanchez, MD

PREOPERATIVE DIAGNOSES
1. Colostomy for obstructing colon cancer.
2. Symptomatic cholelithiasis.

POSTOPERATIVE DIAGNOSES: Same as Preoperative.

PROCEDURES PERFORMED
1. Takedown colostomy with end-to-end colorectostomy.
2. Open cholecystectomy.

ANESTHESIA: General.

PROCEDURE: The patient was brought to the operating room, placed under general anesthesia, and prepped and draped sterilely. The previous midline was reopened with the #10 blade, and we excised the old scar. We carried our dissection through subcutaneous tissues using electrocautery. Midline fascia was divided sharply. We entered the peritoneal cavity and entered the midline fascia along the length of the incision. We took down numerous filmy adhesions and ran the small bowel from the terminal ileum to the ligament of Treitz, which appeared normal. First, we placed an Omni retractor and exposed the right upper quadrant. We identified the cystic duct and cystic artery and tied them off with 0 silk ties distally before transecting them. We then shelled the gallbladder from its fossa using electrocautery. We placed a pack up by the liver bed. We then identified the rectal stump and dissected this free. We then made an elliptical incision around the colostomy opening and carried our dissection down to fascia, freed up the stoma, and fired our TLC 75 stapler across the descending colon. We then sent the specimen to pathology for permanent. We mobilized the left colon along the avascular line of Toldt up and around the splenic flexure. Once we had adequate length we placed a Glassman clamp proximally on the rectum and distally on the descending colon. We then performed a two-layer, hand-sewn, end-to-end anastomosis with an outer layer of 3–0 silk Lembert and inner layer of running 3–0 Vicryl. There was a patent anastomosis, and we could easily milk contents through with no evidence of spilling. We then closed the fascia from the colostomy site with interrupted 0 Vicryl and running 0 PDS. We closed the skin with skin clips.

All sponge and needle counts were correct. The patient tolerated the procedure well and was taken to recovery in stable condition.

CPT Code(s): ______________________________

ICD-10-CM Code(s): ______________________________

ICD-9-CM Code(s): ______________________________

Abstracting Questions

1. What was the approach? ______________________________
2. What did the surgeon do with the existing colostomy? ______________________________
3. What did the surgeon do with the intestinal opening left by removal of the colostomy? ______________________________
4. What type of diagnosis code was reported for the resection of the colostomy? ______________________________
5. What is the stoma? ______________________________

Case 18-9: Modified Radical Mastectomy

LOCATION: Inpatient, Hospital

PATIENT: Lucy Bates

ATTENDING PHYSICIAN: Gary Sanchez, MD

SURGEON: Gary Sanchez, MD

PREOPERATIVE DIAGNOSIS: Right breast cancer.

POSTOPERATIVE DIAGNOSIS: Right breast cancer.

PROCEDURE PERFORMED: Right modified radical mastectomy.

ANESTHESIA: General.

PROCEDURE: The patient was brought to the operating room, placed under general anesthesia, and prepped and draped sterilely. An elliptical incision was made around the right nipple to include the biopsy site, and flaps were created superiorly, inferiorly, medially, and laterally down to the pectoralis superiorly to the rectus fascia inferiorly, sternum medially, and latissimus laterally. We then took the breast off the pectoralis fascia and entered the axillary space. Perforating vessels were either cauterized or ligated with 3–0 Vicryl suture ligatures. We entered the axillary space. We could feel several lymph nodes. We took the lymph nodes. We could see the thoracodorsal nerve easily and kept this free from our dissection. We were unable to identify the long thoracic nerve. Once we had stripped the lymph nodes free, we irrigated with saline. We could easily see the axillary vein superiorly, the latissimus dorsi laterally, and the pectoralis medially and had cleaned all the lymph nodes out of this space. We then irrigated with sterile water and placed two Jackson-Pratt drains, a lateral drain going into the axilla and a medial drain going underneath the skin flaps. We then closed in two layers with a deep layer of 3–0 Vicryl. Steri-Strips and sterile Band-Aids were applied.

All sponge and needle counts were correct. The patient tolerated the procedure well and was taken to recovery in stable condition.

CPT Code(s): ______________________________

ICD-10-CM Code(s): ______________________________

ICD-9-CM Code(s): ______________________________

Abstracting Questions

1. Was this a radical mastectomy? ______________________________
2. Was lymph node dissection reported separately? ______________________________
3. Was skin grafting performed? ______________________________

Case 18-10: Incision and Drainage of Perirectal Abscess

LOCATION: Outpatient, Hospital

PATIENT: Suzy Tarsinski

ATTENDING PHYSICIAN: Gary Sanchez, MD

SURGEON: Gary Sanchez, MD

PREOPERATIVE DIAGNOSIS: Perirectal abscess.

POSTOPERATIVE DIAGNOSIS: Perirectal abscess.

PROCEDURE PERFORMED: Incision and drainage of perirectal abscess.

PROCEDURE: The patient was brought back to the operating room, and after a spinal anesthetic had been given, the area of the rectum was cleaned and draped in the usual fashion after the patient had been placed in a jackknife position. An incision was made over the top of this abscess with a #10-blade scalpel. We entered the abscessed cavity, which returned large amounts of purulent material. We broke up the loculations, debrided the necrotic tissue with a #10 blade, and irrigated with a liter of saline. We then were able to pack the cavity with sewed Kerlix. The patient tolerated the procedure well, and at the end of the procedure all sponges and needles were accounted for. She could soon be transferred to the Post Anesthesia Care Unit in stable condition.

CPT Code(s): ______________________________

ICD-10-CM Code(s): ______________________________

ICD-9-CM Code(s): ______________________________

Abstracting Questions

1. In what subsection within the Surgery section of the CPT will the code to report this service be located?

   ____

2. Does the location of the abscess affect CPT code assignment? ______________________________
3. The report states, "patient was brought back to the operating room." Was a modifier required to report the current services based on that statement? ______________________________

Case 18-11: Peritoneal Dialysis Catheter Placement

OPERATIVE REPORT

LOCATION: Inpatient, Hospital

PATIENT: Gordon Whitefield

ATTENDING PHYSICIAN: Gary Sanchez, MD

PRIMARY CARE PHYSICIAN: George Orbitz, MD

SURGEON: Gary Sanchez, MD

PREOPERATIVE DIAGNOSIS: End-stage renal disease.

POSTOPERATIVE DIAGNOSIS: End-stage renal disease.

PROCEDURE PERFORMED: Peritoneal dialysis catheter placement, tunneled.

INDICATION: Gordon is a 75-year-old male who has end-stage renal disease. I met with him and with his wife three separate times to discuss placement of peritoneal dialysis catheter. We discussed all of this in detail as well as the risks involved. They understood and wished to proceed. Dr. Orbitz said the patient will need to be on peritoneal dialysis. He would like to be able to start this soon. This is because of rhabdomyolysis. We will try to get this watertight so that it can be used tomorrow.

PROCEDURE: The patient was brought to the operating theater and placed in the supine position on the operating table. After receiving some IV sedation, he was prepped and draped in a sterile fashion. A vertical incision line below the umbilicus was infiltrated with 0.5% Marcaine with epinephrine. We waited a few minutes. Incision was made. Dissection was carried sharply down through the subcutaneous tissues to the anterior fascia. The anterior fascia was divided. We then divided the posterior fascia. We then were able to grasp the peritoneum in a three-step technique and then entered the peritoneal cavity sharply. A Tenckhoff catheter was coiled up on the Bozeman catheter and inserted into the peritoneal cavity and down into the pelvis. This went in quite easily. We then used a 3–0 Vicryl to close the peritoneum in a pursestring fashion around the bottom of the cuff. We had two bites that also incorporated this into the cuff to make sure it was secured well. We then likewise did this to the posterior fascia again. This was to help give it more security and a better watertight seal. We then closed the anterior fascia with interrupted sutures of 0 Vicryl in a figure-of-eight fashion. We flushed the catheter out with heparinized saline. This flushed in easily and drained out well. We then created a tunnel. We had marked this out with a marking pen and had previously anesthetized this all with 0.5% Marcaine with epinephrine. A counter incision site was made in the left lower quadrant. Using a Kelly clamp, we made a tract for the tunnel. We then tunneled the catheter through this. The second cuff was in the subcutaneous tissues here. We closed the subcutaneous tissues around the catheter. We closed the skin with a 4–0 Vicryl in a subcuticular fashion. Steri-Strips and sterile dressing were applied. The catheter worked well at the end of the procedure. We flushed this out easily, and it drained back well.

The patient went to the recovery room in stable condition. I met with the patient's wife postoperatively and discussed the operative case.

CPT Code(s): ______________________________

ICD-10-CM Code(s): ______________________________

ICD-9-CM Code(s): ______________________________

Abstracting Questions

1. Does the approach for insertion of the catheter affect code assignment? ______________________________
2. Does the temporary status of the catheter affect the code assignment? ______________________________

Appendix

Coding Answers to Patient Cases

CHAPTER 1: EVALUATION AND MANAGEMENT

Case 1-1
Professional Service: 99238 (Evaluation and Management, Hospital, Discharge)
ICD-10-CM: R07.89 (Pain, chest, non-cardiac)

ICD-9-CM: 786.59 (Pain, chest, non-cardiac)

Case 1-2
Professional Service: 99232 (Evaluation and Management, Hospital)

ICD-10-CM: N17.9 (Failure, renal, acute), **I12.9** (Hypertension, kidney, with stage I through stage IV chronic kidney disease), **N18.9** (Failure, renal, chronic), **E86.9** (Depletion, volume NOS), **I73.9** (Disease, vascular, peripheral [occlusive])

ICD-9-CM: 584.9 (Failure, renal, acute), **403.90** (Hypertension, kidney, with chronic kidney disease, unspecified), **585.9** (Failure, renal, chronic), **276.50** (Depletion, volume), **443.9** (Disease, vascular, peripheral)

Case 1-3
Professional Service: 99232 (Hospital Services, Inpatient Services, Subsequent Hospital Care)

ICD-10-CM: T46.5x5A (Antihypertensive drug NEC, Adverse Effect), **I95.2** (Hypotension, orthostatic [chronic], due to drugs), **E86.9** (Depletion, volume NOS), **R07.9** (Pain, chest), **Z99.2** (Dependence, on, renal dialysis [peritoneal])

ICD-9-CM: 458.0 (Hypotension, orthostatic), **276.50** (Depletion, volume), **786.50** (Pain, chest), **E942.6** (Antihypertensive agents NEC, External Cause [E Code], Therapeutic), **V45.11** (Status, dialysis [peritoneal])

Case 1-4
Professional Service: 99239 (Hospital Services, Inpatient Services, Discharge Services)

ICD-10-CM: I12.9 (Hypertension, kidney, with stage I through stage IV chronic kidney disease), **N18.9** (Failure, renal, chronic), **E11.22** (Diabetes, diabetic, type 2, with, chronic kidney disease)

ICD-9-CM: 403.90 (Hypertension, kidney, with chronic kidney disease, Unspecified), **585.9** (Failure, renal, chronic), **250.40** (Diabetes, diabetic, with nephropathy), **583.81** (Nephropathy, diabetic)

Case 1-5
Professional Service: 99243 (Consultation, Office and/or Other Outpatient)

ICD-10-CM: I10 (Hypertension), **I73.9** (Disease, vascular, peripheral [occlusive])

ICD-9-CM: 401.9 (Hypertension, Unspecified), **443.9** (Disease, vascular, peripheral)

Case 1-6
Professional Service: 99242 (Consultation, Office and/or Other Outpatient)

ICD-10-CM: I12.9 (Hypertension, kidney, with, stage I through stage IV chronic kidney disease), **N18.9** (Failure, renal, chronic), **D64.9** (Anemia)

ICD-9-CM: 403.90 (Hypertension, kidney, with chronic kidney disease, Unspecified), **585.9** (Failure, renal, chronic), **285.9** (Anemia)

Case 1-7
Professional Service: 99238 (Hospital Services, Inpatient Services, Discharge Services)

ICD-10-CM: M10.022 (Gout, idiopathic, elbow, left elbow), **E11.52** (Diabetes, with, gangrene), **E11.22** (Diabetes with chronic kidney disease), **N18.6** (Disease, renal, end-stage [failure]), **Z99.2** (Status, dialysis [hemodialysis])

ICD-9-CM: 274.00 (Gout, arthritis), **250.70** (Diabetes, with gangrene), **785.4** (Gangrene), **250.40** (Diabetes with nephropathy), **583.81** (Nephropathy, in diabetes), **585.6** (Disease, renal, end-stage), **V45.11** (Status, dialysis)

Case 1-8
Professional Service: 99238 (Hospital Services, Inpatient Services, Discharge Services)

ICD-10-CM: N17.9 (Failure, renal, acute), **I12.9** (Hypertension, kidney, with, stage I through stage IV chronic kidney disease), **N18.9** (Failure, renal, chronic), **K21.9** (Reflux, esophageal), **J45.909** (Asthma, unspecified)

ICD-9-CM: 584.9 (Failure, renal, acute), **403.90** (Hypertension, kidney, with chronic kidney disease, unspecified), **585.9** (Failure, renal, chronic), **530.81** (Reflux, esophageal), **493.90** (Asthma, unspecified)

Case 1-9
Professional Service: 99231 (Hospital Services, Inpatient Services, Subsequent Hospital Care)

ICD-10-CM: R04.2 (Hemoptysis), **J96.9** (Failure, respiration, respiratory)

ICD-9-CM: 786.39 (Hemoptysis), **518.81** (Failure, respiratory)

Case 1-10
Professional Service: 99252 (Consultation, Inpatient)

ICD-10-CM: S06.0x9A (Concussion [brain] [cerebral] [current]), **V47.52xA** (Accident, transport, car occupant, driver, non-collision accident [traffic])

ICD-9-CM: 850.5 (Concussion, with loss of consciousness, unspecified duration), **E816.0** (Collision, motor vehicle, after leaving, running off public highway)

Case 1-11
Professional Service: 99253 (Consultation, Inpatient)

ICD-10-CM: S16.9xxA (Injury, muscle, neck [level]), **W18.39xA** (Fall, same level), **Y93.43** (Activity [involving], gymnastics)

ICD-9-CM: 959.09 (Injury, neck), **E888.8** (Fall, other), **E005.2** (Index to External Causes, Activity, gymnastics)

Case 1-12
Professional Service: 99252 (Consultation, Inpatient)

ICD-10-CM: M51.16 (Displacement, intervertebral disk, lumbar region, with, neuritis, radiculitis, radiculopathy or sciatica)

ICD-9-CM: 722.10 (Displacement, intervertebral disk, lumbar)

Case 1-13
Professional Service: No charge

ICD-10-CM: I61.1 (Hemorrhage, intracranial [nontraumatic], intracerebral [nontraumatic] [in], hemisphere, cortical)

ICD-9-CM: 431 (Hematoma, brain, nontraumatic)

Case 1-14
Professional Service: 99253 (Consultation, Inpatient)

ICD-10-CM: R53.1 (Asthenia), **M54.6** (Pain, spine, thoracic), **M54.5** (Pain, lumbar region), **I25.10** (Disease, heart, ischemic, atherosclerotic), **J44.9** (Disease, pulmonary, chronic obstructive), **I10** (Hypertension)

ICD-9-CM: 780.9 (Weakness), **724.1** (Pain, thoracic), **724.2** (Pain, lumbar), **414.9** (Disease, coronary), **496** (Obstruction, airway, chronic), **427.31** (Fibrillation, atrial), **401.9** (Hypertension)

Case 1-15
Professional Service: 99253 (Consultation, Inpatient)

ICD-10-CM: N13.30 (Hydronephrosis, NEC), **N27.0** (Small, kidney, unknown cause, unilateral)

ICD-9-CM: 591 (Hydronephrosis), **589.0** (Small, kidney, unknown cause, unilateral)

Case 1-16
Professional Service: 99231 (Evaluation and Management, Hospital)

ICD-10-CM: C34.2 (Neoplasm, lung middle lobe, right side, Malignant, Primary), **J44.9** (Disease, pulmonary, chronic obstructive)

ICD-9-CM: 162.4 (Neoplasm, lung middle lobe, Malignant, Primary), **493.20** (Disease, pulmonary, obstructive diffuse, with asthma, unspecified)

Case 1-17
Professional Service: 99214 (Evaluation and Management, Office and Other Outpatient)

ICD-10-CM: A08.4 (Gastroenteritis, viral NEC)

ICD-9-CM: 008.8 (Gastroenteritis, viral NEC)

Case 1-18
Professional Service: 99242 (Consultation, Office or Outpatient)

ICD-10-CM: R07.9 (Pain, chest), **R06.02** (Shortness, breath)

ICD-9-CM: 786.50 (Pain, chest), **786.05** (Shortness, breath)

Case 1-19
Professional Service: 99214 (Evaluation and Management, Office and Other Outpatient)

ICD-10-CM: R10.31 (Pain, abdominal, lower, right quadrant)

ICD-9-CM: 789.03 (Pain, abdominal)

CHAPTER 2: ANESTHESIOLOGY

Case 2-1
Professional Service: 00840-QK-P2 (Anesthesia, Abdomen, Intraperitoneal), **99100** (Anesthesia, Special Circumstances, Extreme Age)

Case 2-2
Professional Service: 00830-QK-P2 (Anesthesia, Abdomen, Hernia Repair)

Case 2-3
Professional Service: 00790-AA-P3 (Anesthesia, Laparoscopy, Upper Abdomen)

Case 2-4
Professional Service: 00400-AA-QS-P1 (Anesthesia, Integumentary System, Anterior Trunk)

Case 2-5
Professional Service: 01232-AA-P3 (Anesthesia, Leg, Upper)

Case 2-6
Professional Service: 00750-AA-P1 (Anesthesia, Hernia Repair, Abdomen, Upper)

Case 2-7
Professional Service: 00790-QK-P2 (Anesthesia, Abdomen, Intraperitoneal)

Case 2-8
Professional Service: 00404-AA-P1 (Anesthesia, Breast)

Case 2-9
Professional Service: 00902-AA-P3 (Anesthesia, Anus)

Case 2-10
Professional Service: 00400-AA-P2 (Anesthesia, Integumentary System, Hand)

Case 2-11
Professional Service: 00211-AA-P5 (Anesthesia, Brain)

CHAPTER 3: CARDIOLOGY

Case 3-1
Professional Service: 36556 (Venous Access Device, Insertion, Central)

ICD-10-CM: E87.7 (Overload, fluid), **N17.9** (Failure, renal, acute)

ICD-9-CM: 276.69 (Overload, fluid), **584.9** (Failure, renal, acute)

Case 3-2
Professional Service: 36514 (Apheresis, Therapeutic)

ICD-10-CM: G70.00 (Myasthenia, gravis)

ICD-9-CM: 358.00 (Myasthenia, gravis)

Case 3-3
Professional Service: 36557 (Vein, Catheterization, Central Insertion)

ICD-10-CM: N00.7 (Glomerulonephritis, crescentic)

ICD-9-CM: 580.4 (Glomerulonephritis, necrotizing, acute)

Case 3-4
Professional Service: 33533 (Coronary Artery Bypass, Arterial), **33517** (Coronary Artery Bypass Graft, Arterial-Venous)

ICD-10-CM: I25.110 (Arteriosclerosis, coronary [artery], native vessel, with, angina pectoris, unstable)

ICD-9-CM: 414.01 (Arteriosclerosis, coronary, native artery), **411.1** (Angina, accelerated)

Case 3-5
Professional Service: 31500 (Insertion, Endotracheal Tube, Emergency Intubation)

ICD-10-CM: J96.0 (Failure, respiration/respiratory, acute)

ICD-9-CM: 518.81 (Failure, respiration/respiratory, acute)

Case 3-6
Professional Service: 35800 (Exploration, Blood Vessel, Neck)

ICD-10-CM: J95.01 (Complications, tracheostomy, hemorrhage), **C94.6** (Disease, myeloproliferative, not classified)

ICD-9-CM: 519.09 (Tracheostomy, hemorrhage), **238.79** (Disorder, myeloproliferative, NEC)

Case 3-7
Professional Service: 32400-LT (Biopsy, Pleura, Needle)

ICD-10-CM: J90 (Effusion, pleura)

ICD-9-CM: 511.9 (Effusion, pleura)

Case 3-8
Professional Service: 35301-LT (Thromboendarterectomy, Carotid Artery), **95955-26** (Electroencephalography (EEG), Intraoperative)

ICD-10-CM: I65.22 (Occlusion, artery, carotid)

ICD-9-CM: 433.10 (Arteriosclerosis, carotid)

Case 3-9
Professional Service: 36217-RT (Insertion, Catheter, Brachiocephalic Artery), **36216-59-51-LT** (Insertion, Catheter, Brachiocephalic Artery), **36215-59-51-LT** (Insertion, Catheter, Brachiocephalic Artery)

ICD-10-CM: I61.1 (Hemorrhage, intracranial [non-traumatic], intracerebral, hemisphere, cortical [superficial])

ICD-9-CM: 431 (Hemorrhage, intracerebral)

Case 3-10
Professional Service: 33967 (Insertion, Balloon, Intra-aortic)

ICD-10-CM: I25.10 (Arteriosclerosis, coronary [artery], native vessel)

ICD-9-CM: 414.01 (Arteriosclerosis, coronary [artery], native artery)

CHAPTER 4: INTEGUMENTARY

Case 4-1
Professional Service: 11312 (Lesion, Skin, Shaving)

ICD-10-CM: D23.39 (Neoplasm, skin, cheek, Benign)

ICD-9-CM: 216.3 (Neoplasm, skin, cheek [external], Benign)

Case 4-2
Professional Service: 19120-RT (Breast, Excision, Lesion)

ICD-10-CM: C50.011 (Neoplasm, breast, female, nipple, Malignant Primary)

ICD-9-CM: 174.0 (Neoplasm, breast, nipple, Malignant, Primary)

Case 4-3
Professional Service: 15574-F7 (Pedicle Flap, Formation), **15120-51** (Split, Grafts)

ICD-10-CM: S68.622A (Amputation, traumatic, finger, transphalangeal, partial, middle), **W31.9xxA** (External Cause Index, Contact with, machinery)

ICD-9-CM: 886.0 (Amputation, finger), **E919.9** (Index to External Cause Accident, caused by, machinery, unspecified)

Case 4-4
Professional Service: 15620-58-F7 (Skin Graft and Flap, Delay of Flap)

ICD-10-CM: Z47.81 (Aftercare, following surgery [for] [on], amputation), **Z89.021** (Absence, finger[s] [acquired])

ICD-9-CM: V54.89 (Aftercare, amputation stump), **V49.62** (Absence, finger)

Case 4-5
Professional Service: 12002-F7 (Closure)

ICD-10-CM: S61.202A (Laceration, finger[s], middle, right), **W45.8xxA** (External Cause Index, Contact [accidental] with, arrow, not thrown, projected or falling)

ICD-9-CM: 883.0 (Wound, open, finger, with tendon involvement), **E920.8** (Index to External Causes, Cut, by, arrow)

Case 4-6
Professional Service: 49060-78-52 (Drainage, Abscess, Retroperitoneal), **11005-78-51** (Debridement, Skin, Subcutaneous Tissue, Infected)

ICD-10-CM: T81.4xxD (Infection, postoperative wound), **K65.4** (Necrosis, fat, peritoneum), **I96** (Necrosis, skin or subcutaneous tissue), **K63.2** (Fistula, abdominal wall)

ICD-9-CM: 998.59 (Infection, postoperative wound), **567.82** (Necrosis, fat, fatty [generalized], abdominal wall) or (Necrosis, peritoneum), **709.3** (Necrosis, skin [subcutaneous]), **569.81** (Fistula, abdominal wall)

Case 4-7
Professional Service: 11005-58 (Debridement, Skin, Subcutaneous Tissue, Infected)

ICD-10-CM: K65.4 (Necrosis, fat, abdominal wall), **I96** (Necrosis, skin or subcutaneous tissue NEC), **T81.83xD** (Fistula, postoperative, persistent)

ICD-9-CM: 567.82 (Necrosis, fat, abdominal wall), **709.8** (Necrosis, skin [subcutaneous tissue]), **998.6** (Fistula, postoperative, persistent)

Case 4-8
Professional Service: 26952-54-F7 (Tissue, Transfer, Adjacent, Skin)

ICD-10-CM: S68.622A (Amputation, traumatic, finger, transphalangeal, partial, middle), **W23.0xxA** (External Cause Index, Crushed, between objects)

ICD-9-CM: 886.0 (Amputation, finger), **E918** (Index to External Causes, Crushed, between objects)

Case 4-9
Professional Service: 11404-58 (Excision, Skin, Lesion, Benign)

ICD-10-CM: D23.61 (Neoplasm, skin, arm, Benign)

ICD-9-CM: 216.6 (Neoplasm, skin, arm, Benign)

CHAPTER 5: EMERGENCY MEDICINE

Case 5-1
Professional Service: 99281 (Evaluation and Management, Emergency Department)

ICD-10-CM: S50.11xA (Contusion, forearm), **S50.811A** (Abrasion, forearm), **W21.9xxA** (Index to External Causes, Struck by, object, thrown, in sports), **Y92.211** (External Cause Index, Place of occurrence, school, elementary school), **Y93.22** (External Cause Index, Activity [involving], ice, hockey)

ICD-9-CM: 923.10 (Contusion, forearm), **913.0** (Injury, superficial, forearm), **E917.0** (Index to External Causes, Hit, other person, in sports), **E849.6** (Accident, occurring at, school), **E003.1** (Index to External Causes, Activity, Hockey)

Case 5-2
Professional Service: 99284 (Emergency Department Services)

ICD-10-CM: R11.2 (Vomiting, with nausea), **E86.0** (Dehydration), **C15.9** (Neoplasm, esophagus, Malignant Primary), **C79.51** (Neoplasm, bones, Malignant Secondary), **C78.89** (Neoplasm, stomach, Malignant Secondary)

ICD-9-CM: 787.01 (Vomiting, with nausea), **276.51** (Dehydration), **150.9** (Neoplasm, esophagus, Malignant, Primary), **198.5** (Neoplasm, bones, Malignant, Secondary), **197.8** (Neoplasm, stomach, Malignant, Secondary)

Case 5-3
Professional Service: 99284 (Emergency Department Services)

ICD-10-CM: R50.9 (Fever), **R11.2** (Nausea with vomiting), **E86.0** (Dehydration), **R79.1** (Prolonged, bleeding [time])

ICD-9-CM: 780.60 (Fever), **787.01** (Nausea with vomiting), **276.51** (Dehydration), **790.92** (Prolonged, bleeding time)

Case 5-4
Professional Service: 99284 (Emergency Department Services)

ICD-10-CM: I60.9 (Hemorrhage, intracranial, subarachnoid [nontraumatic])

ICD-9-CM: 430 (Hemorrhage, subarachnoid, nontraumatic)

Case 5-5
Professional Service: 99284 (Evaluation and Management, Emergency Department)

ICD-10-CM: S06.0x0A (Concussion [brain] [cerebral] [current]), **W17.82xA** (External Cause Index, Fall, from, one level to another), **Y92.512** (External Cause Index, Place of occurrence, store)

ICD-9-CM: 850.0 (Concussion without loss of consciousness), **E884.9** (Index to External Causes, Fall, from, one, level to another), **E849.6** (Index to External Causes, Accident, occurring, store)

Case 5-6
Professional Service: 99282 (Evaluation and Management, Emergency Department)

ICD-10-CM: H66.92 (Otitis, media, acute, subacute, viral NEC), **J06.9** (Infection, respiratory, upper [acute])

ICD-9-CM: 382.9 (Otitis, media, acute), **465.9** (Infection, respiratory, upper, acute)

Case 5-7
Professional Service: 99284 (Evaluation and Management, Emergency Department)

ICD-10-CM: L03.115 (Cellulitis, lower limb)

ICD-9-CM: 682.6 (Cellulitis, leg)

Case 5-8
Professional Service: 99282 (Evaluation and Management, Emergency Department)

ICD-10-CM: S83.005A (Dislocation, patella, left), **Y93.67** (External Cause Index, Activity, [involving], basketball), **Y92.838** (Place of occurrence, recreation area)

ICD-9-CM: 836.3 (Dislocation, patella), **E007.6** (Index to External Causes, Activity, basketball), **E849.4** (Accident [to], occurring [at] [in], place, recreational)

Case 5-9
Professional Service: 99281 (Evaluation and Management, Emergency Department Services)

ICD-10-CM: S81.812A (Laceration, leg [lower], left), **W45.8xxA** (External Cause Index, Contact with, object, sharp NEC)

ICD-9-CM: 891.1 (Wound, open, leg, complicated), **E920.9** (Index to External Causes, Cut, cutting)

Case 5-10
Professional Service: 99284 (Evaluation and Management, Emergency Department)

ICD-10-CM: R19.7 (Diarrhea), **R10.9** (Pain, abdominal)

ICD-9-CM: 787.91 (Diarrhea), **789.00** (Pain, abdominal)

Case 5-11
Professional Service: 99281 (Evaluation and Management, Emergency Department)

ICD-10-CM: I86.1 (Varicose, scrotum)

ICD-9-CM: 456.4 (Varicose [ulcerated], scrotum)

Case 5-12
Professional Service: 99284 (Evaluation and Management, Emergency Department)

ICD-10-CM: R06.00 (Dyspnea), **R00.0** (Tachycardia), **I25.2** (History, personal, myocardial infarction [old]), **Z95.1** (Status, aortocoronary bypass)

ICD-9-CM: 786.09 (Dyspnea), **785.0** (Tachycardia), **412** (Infarction, myocardium, healed or old), **V45.81** (Status, shunt, aortocoronary bypass)

CHAPTER 6: MEDICINE

Case 6-1
Professional Service: 93306-26 (Echocardiography, Cardiac, Transthoracic)

ICD-10-CM: I07.1 (Insufficiency, tricuspid), **I48.0** (Fibrillation, atrial or auricular [established]), **I51.9** (Dysfunction, ventricular)

ICD-9-CM: 397.0 (Insufficiency, tricuspid), **427.31** (Fibrillation, atrial), **429.9** (Dysfunction, ventricular)

Case 6-2
Professional Service: 93016 (Stress Tests, Cardiovascular), **93018** (Stress Tests, Cardiovascular)

ICD-10-CM: Z01.810 (Examination, pre-procedural, cardiovascular), **Z95.2** (Replacement by artificial or mechanical device or prosthesis, heart, valve)

ICD-9-CM: V72.81 (Admission for, examination, preoperative, cardiovascular), **V43.3** (Replacement by artificial or mechanical device or prosthesis, heart, valve)

Case 6-3
Professional Service: 93458-26 (Catheterization, Cardiac, Left Heart)

ICD-10-CM: I25.110 (Arteriosclerosis, coronary [artery], native vessel, with angina pectoris, unstable)

ICD-9-CM: 411.1 (Angina, unstable), **414.01** (Arteriosclerosis, coronary [artery], native artery)

Case 6-4
Professional Service: 93458-26 (Catheterization, Cardiac, Left Heart)

ICD-10-CM: R94.30 (Abnormal, function, studies, cardiovascular), **R06.02** (Shortness, breath)

ICD-9-CM: 794.39 (Abnormal, function studies, cardiovascular), **786.05** (Shortness, breath)

Case 6-5
Professional Service: 93503 (Catheterization, Cardiac, Flow Directed)

ICD-10-CM: E23.2 (Diabetes, insipidus)

ICD-9-CM: 253.5 (Diabetes, insipidus)

Case 6-6
Professional Service: 93965-26 (Doppler Scan, Extremities)

ICD-10-CM: E11.59 (Diabetes, with circulatory complications), **I73.9** (Disease, peripheral, vascular NOS)

ICD-9-CM: 250.00 (Diabetes), **443.9** (Disease, vascular, peripheral [occlusive])

Case 6-7
Professional Service: 93971-26-LT (Duplex Scan, Venous Studies, Extremity)

ICD-10-CM: Z01.810 (Examination, preprocedural, cardiovascular), **I25.10** (Arteriosclerosis, coronary [artery], native vessel), **R07.9** (Pain, chest)

ICD-9-CM: V72.81 (Examination, preprocedural, cardiovascular), **414.01** (Arteriosclerosis, coronary, native artery), **786.50** (Pain, chest)

Case 6-8
Professional Service: 93971-26 (Duplex Scan, Venous Studies, Extremity)

ICD-10-CM: M79.606 (Pain, limb, lower), **M79.89** (Swelling, leg)

ICD-9-CM: 729.5 (Pain, leg), **729.81** (Swelling, leg)

Case 6-9
Professional Service: 93970-26 (Duplex Scan, Venous Studies, Extremity), **76700-26** (Ultrasound, Abdomen)

ICD-10-CM: M79.89 (Swelling, leg), **R06.9** (Abnormal/abnormality/abnormalities, breathing), **R18.8** (Ascites [abdominal])

ICD-9-CM: 729.81 (Swelling, leg), **786.09** (Breathing, labored), **789.59** (Ascites)

Case 6-10
Professional Service: 90966 (Dialysis, End Stage Renal Disease)

ICD-10-CM: N18.6 (Disease, renal, end-stage), **D63.1** (Anemia, in, end stage renal disease)

ICD-9-CM: 585.6 (Disease, renal, end-stage), **285.21** (Anemia, in, end-stage renal disease [failure])

CHAPTER 7: GASTROENTEROLOGY

Case 7-1
Professional Service: 43752 (Placement, Orogastric Tube)

ICD-10-CM: K31.89 (Gastroparesis)

ICD-9-CM: 536.3 (Paresis, stomach)

Case 7-2
Professional Service: 44143 (Hartmann Procedure), **44139** (Mobilization, Splenic Flexure), **38102** (Splenectomy, Total, En bloc), **47001** (Biopsy, Liver), **32551-59-51-RT** (Thoracostomy, Tube)

ICD-10-CM: K63.1 (Perforation, intestine), **C94.6** (Disease, myeloproliferative, not classified), **J90** (Effusion, pleura), **A41.9** (Sepsis, unspecified)

ICD-9-CM: 569.83 (Perforation, intestine), **238.79** (Disorder, myeloproliferative [chronic]), **511.9** (Effusion, pleura), **038.9** (Septicemia), **995.91** (Sepsis)

Case 7-3
Professional Service: 49440 (Gastrostomy Tube, Placement, Percutaneous, Nonendoscopic), **49446-51** (Gastrostomy Tube, Conversion to Gastro-jejunostomy Tube), **76942-26** (Ultrasound, Needle or Catheter Placement)

ICD-10-CM: E46 (Malnutrition)

ICD-9-CM: 263.9 (Malnutrition)

Case 7-4
Professional Service: 49000-78 (Laparotomy, Exploration)

ICD-10-CM: N99.72 (Complication, intraoperative, puncture or laceration [accidental], genitourinary organ or structure, during procedure on other organ)

ICD-9-CM: 998.2 (Puncture, accidental, complicating surgery)

Case 7-5
Professional Service: 44640-22 (Repair, Intestines, Small, Fistula), **44120-51** (Excision, Intestines, Small)

ICD-10-CM: K63.2 (Fistula, intestine)

ICD-9-CM: 569.81 (Fistula, intestine)

Case 7-6
Professional Service: 43117-62 (Esophagectomy, Partial), **47100** (Biopsy, Liver), **47000-59-53-51** (Biopsy, Liver), **44015** (Jejunostomy, Insertion, Catheter)

ICD-10-CM: K22.711 (Barrett's esophagus, with dysplasia, high grade), **D18.03** (Hemangioma, intra-abdominal)

ICD-9-CM: 530.85 (Barrett's esophagus), **228.04** (Hemangioma, intra-abdominal structures)

CHAPTER 8: NEPHROLOGY

Case 8-1
Professional Service: 99231 (Evaluation and Management, Hospital)

ICD-10-CM: N17.9 (Failure, renal, acute), **I12.9** (Hypertension, kidney, stage I through stage IV chronic kidney disease), **N18.9** (Failure, renal, chronic), **R60.0** (Edema, legs)

ICD-9-CM: 584.9 (Failure, renal, acute), **403.90** (Hypertension, kidney, with chronic kidney disease, unspecified), **585.9** (Failure, renal, chronic), **782.3** (Edema)

Case 8-2
Professional Service: 90945 (Dialysis, Peritoneal)

ICD-10-CM: N18.6 (Disease, renal, end-stage), **E11.40** (Diabetes, with, nephropathy)

ICD-9-CM: 585.6 (Disease, renal, end-stage), **250.40** (Diabetes, with nephropathy), **583.81** (Nephropathy, with diabetes)

Case 8-3
Professional Service: 90947 (Dialysis, Peritoneal)

ICD-10-CM: N18.6 (Disease, renal, end-stage)

ICD-9-CM: 585.6 (Disease, renal, end-stage)

Case 8-4
Professional Service: 50280-RT (Excision, Cyst, Kidney)

ICD-10-CM: N28.1 (Cyst, kidney [acquired])

ICD-9-CM: 593.2 (Cyst, kidney, acquired)

Case 8-5
Professional Service: 50541-RT (Kidney, Cyst, Ablation)

ICD-10-CM: N28.1 (Cyst, kidney [acquired])

ICD-9-CM: 593.2 (Cyst, kidney, acquired)

Case 8-6
Professional Service: 50205-LT (Biopsy, Kidney)

ICD-10-CM: N28.1 (Cyst, kidney [acquired])

ICD-9-CM: 593.2 (Cyst, kidney, acquired)

Case 8-7
Professional Service: 36580 (Vein, Catheterization, Replacement)

ICD-10-CM: Z49.01 (Preparatory care for subsequent treatment NEC, for dialysis), **N18.6** (Disease, renal, end stage)

ICD-9-CM: V56.1 (Admission for dialysis, catheter removal or replacement), **585.6** (Disease, renal, end stage)

CHAPTER 9: NEUROLOGY AND OPHTHALMOLOGY

Case 9-1
Professional Service: 61313-RT (Craniotomy, Surgery)

ICD-10-CM: I61.1 (Hemorrhage, intracranial [nontraumatic], intracerebral, hemisphere, cortical [superficial])

ICD-9-CM: 431 (Hematoma, brain, nontraumatic)

Case 9-2
Professional Service: 64718-LT (Neuroplasty, Peripheral Nerve)

ICD-10-CM: G56.22 (Palsy, ulnar nerve, [tardy])

ICD-9-CM: 354.2 (Palsy, ulnar nerve, tardy)

Case 9-3
Professional Service: 61154-RT (Burr Hole, Skull, Drainage, Hematoma)

ICD-10-CM: I62.01 (Hemorrhage, intracranial [nontraumatic], subdural [nontraumatic], acute)

ICD-9-CM: 432.1 (Hematoma, subdural, nontraumatic)

Case 9-4
Professional Service: 63030-RT (Hemilaminectomy), **63035-RT** (Hemilaminectomy, each additional space)

ICD-10-CM: M51.27 (Displacement, intervertebral disc, lumbosacral region)

ICD-9-CM: 722.10 (Displacement, intervertebral disc, lumbar, lumbosacral)

Case 9-5
Professional Service: 64721-LT (Carpal Tunnel Syndrome, Decompression)

ICD-10-CM: G56.02 (Syndrome, carpal tunnel)

ICD-9-CM: 354.0 (Carpal tunnel syndrome)

Case 9-6
Professional Service: 63709-78 (Repair, Spinal Cord, Cerebrospinal Fluid Leak)

ICD-10-CM: G97.82 (Pseudomeningocele, postprocedural [spinal])

ICD-9-CM: 997.01 (Pseudomeningocele, postprocedural)

Case 9-7
Professional Service: 63047 (Laminectomy, with Facetectomy), **63048 × 2** (Laminectomy, with Facetectomy)

ICD-10-CM: M48.06 (Stenosis, spinal, lumbar), **M43.16** (Spondylolisthesis, lumbar region)

ICD-9-CM: 724.02 (Stenosis, spinal, lumbar, lumbosacral), **738.4** (Spondylolisthesis, acquired)

Case 9-8
Professional Service: 63042-LT (Hemilaminectomy), **22840** (Insertion, Spinal Instrumentation, Posterior Nonsegmental, Harrington Rod Technique), **22612-51** (Arthrodesis, Vertebra, Lumbar, Posterior/Posterolateral and/or Lateral Transverse Process), **61783** (Stereotaxis, Computer Assisted, Spine Procedure), **95927-26** (Evoked Potential, Somatosensory Testing)

ICD-10-CM: M43.17 (Spondylolisthesis, lumbosacral region)

ICD-9-CM: 738.4 (Spondylolisthesis, acquired)

Case 9-9
Professional Service: 20661 (Halo, Cranial)

ICD-10-CM: S14.104A (Injury, spinal [cord], cervical, C4), **V86.39xA** (External Cause Index, Accident, transport, motor vehicle NEC occupant)

ICD-9-CM: 952.00 (Injury, spinal [cord], cervical [C1-C4]), **952.05** (Injury, spinal cord, cervical, C5-C7 level), **E819.9** (Index to External Causes, Accident, motor vehicle)

Case 9-10
Professional Service: 66984-RT (Removal, Cataract, Extracapsular)

ICD-10-CM: H25.041 (Cataract, senile, subcapsular polar, posterior)

ICD-9-CM: 366.14 (Cataract, senile, posterior subcapsular polar)

CHAPTER 10: OBSTETRICS AND GYNECOLOGY

Case 10-1
Professional Service: 58150 (Hysterectomy, Abdominal, Total)

ICD-10-CM: N92.0 (Menorrhagia [primary]), **D25.9** (Fibroid, uterus)

ICD-9-CM: 626.2 (Menorrhagia), **218.9** (Leiomyoma, uterus)

Case 10-2
Professional Service: 58558 (Dilation and Curettage, Hysteroscopy)

ICD-10-CM: N93.8 (Bleeding, uterus, dysfunctional of functional)

ICD-9-CM: 626.8 (Bleeding, uterus, dysfunctional)

Case 10-3
Professional Service: 59515 (Cesarean Delivery, Postpartum Care)

ICD-10-CM: O45.93 (Pregnancy, complicated by, premature separation of placenta, unspecified, third trimester), **O60.14x0** (Pregnancy, complicated by, preterm labor third trimester, with third trimester preterm delivery), **Z37.0** (Outcome of delivery, single, liveborn)

ICD-9-CM: 641.21 (Placenta, separation), **644.21** (Pregnancy, complicated by early onset of delivery [spontaneous]), **V27.0** (Outcome of delivery, single, liveborn)

Case 10-4
Professional Service: 56630-RT (Vulvectomy, Radical)

ICD-10-CM: D07.1 (Neoplasm, labium, majus, Malignant, Ca in situ)

ICD-9-CM: 233.32 (Neoplasm, labia, majora, Malignant, Ca in situ)

Case 10-5
Professional Service: 58558 (Dilation and Curettage, Hysteroscopy)

ICD-10-CM: N92.0 (Menorrhagia), **N84.0** (Polyps, endometrium)

ICD-9-CM: 626.2 (Menorrhagia), **621.0** (Polyps, endometrium)

Case 10-6
Professional Service: 99214-24 (Evaluation and Management, Office and Other Outpatient)

ICD-10-CM: O34.32 (Pregnancy, complicated by, incompetent, cervix), **Z87.51** (History personal [of], obstetric complications, pre-term labor)

ICD-9-CM: 654.63 (Abnormal, cervix, in pregnancy or childbirth), **V13.21** (History (personal) of, obstetric disorder, pre-term labor)

Case 10-7
Professional Service: 59820 (Abortion, Missed, First Trimester)

ICD-10-CM: O02.1 (Abortion, missed)

ICD-9-CM: 632 (Abortion, missed)

Case 10-8
Professional Service: 59514 (Cesarean Delivery, Delivery Only), **58611** (Cesarean Delivery, Tubal Ligation at Time of)

ICD-10-CM: O60.14x0 (Pregnancy, complicated by, preterm labor, third trimester, with third trimester preterm delivery), **O34.21** (Cesarean delivery, previous, affecting management of pregnancy), **Z37.0** (Outcome of delivery, single, liveborn), **Z30.2** (Encounter [for], sterilization)

ICD-9-CM: 644.21 (Premature, labor), **654.21** (Cesarean delivery, previous, affecting management of pregnancy), **V27.0** (Outcome of delivery, single, liveborn), **V25.2** (Sterilization, admission for)

Case 10-9
Professional Service: 59515 (Cesarean Delivery, Postpartum Care)

ICD-10-CM: O45.93 (Pregnancy, complicated by, premature separation of placenta), **Z37.0** (Outcome of delivery, single, liveborn)

ICD-9-CM: 641.21 (Delivery, complicated by, placenta abruptio), **V27.0** (Outcome of delivery, single, liveborn)

Case 10-10
Professional Service: 76815-26 (Ultrasound, Pregnant Uterus)

ICD-10-CM: O45.93 (Abruptio, placentae, third trimester)

ICD-9-CM: 641.23 (Placenta abruptio)

Case 10-11
Professional Service: 49322 (Laparoscopy, Aspiration)

ICD-10-CM: N83.8 (Cyst, paratubal)

ICD-9-CM: 620.8 (Cyst, paratubal)

CHAPTER 11: ORTHOPEDICS

Case 11-1
Professional Service: 29898-RT (Arthroscopy, Surgical, Ankle)

ICD-10-CM: M19.071 (Osteoarthritis, ankle), **M25.771** (Osteophyte, ankle), **M79.9** (Disorder, soft tissue, ankle)

ICD-9-CM: 715.97 (Osteoarthritis), **726.91** (Exostosis, ankle), **729.90** (Disorder, soft tissue)

Case 11-2
Professional Service: 29881-LT (Arthroscopy, Surgical, Knee)

ICD-10-CM: M23.201 (Derangement, knee, meniscus, due to old tear or injury, lateral), **M17.12** (Osteoarthritis, knee)

ICD-9-CM: 717.41 (Tear, meniscus, lateral, bucket handle, old), **715.96** (Osteoarthrosis, (including osteoarthritis) lower leg)

Case 11-3
Professional Service: 29874-LT (Arthroscopy, Surgical, Knee), **29877-59-51** (Arthroscopy, Surgical, Knee)

ICD-10-CM: S83.92xA (Sprain, knee), **M23.42** (Loose, body, joint, knee), **M22.42** (Chondromalacia, knee, patella), **M67.52** (Plica, syndrome, knee)

ICD-9-CM: 844.9 (Sprain, knee), **717.6** (Loose, body, joint, knee), **717.7** (Chondromalacia, patella), **727.83** (Plica, knee)

Case 11-4
Professional Service: 29881-RT (Arthroscopy, Surgical, Knee)

ICD-10-CM: M23.203 (Derangement, knee, meniscus, due to old tear or injury, medial), **M17.11** (Osteoarthritis, knee)

ICD-9-CM: 717.0 (Tear, meniscus, medial, bucket handle, old), **715.96** (Osteoarthrosis, lower leg)

Case 11-5
Professional Service: 20610-LT (Injection, Joint)

ICD-10-CM: M75.52 (Bursitis, shoulder)

ICD-9-CM: 726.19 (Bursitis, subacromial)

Case 11-6
Professional Service: 26746-FA (Metacarpophalangeal Joint, Fracture, Open)

ICD-10-CM: S62.232A (Fracture, traumatic, metacarpal, first, base [displaced]), **X58.xxxA** (External Cause Index, Fracture, circumstances unknown or unspecified)

ICD-9-CM: 815.01 (Fracture, metacarpal, base, thumb, closed), **E887** (Index to External Causes, Fracture, circumstances unknown or unspecified)

Case 11-7
Professional Service: 25210-LT (Carpal Bone, Excision), **25310-51-LT** (Tendon, Transfer, Wrist)

ICD-10-CM: M18.12 (Osteoarthritis, hand joint, first carpometacarpal joint)

ICD-9-CM: 715.94 (Osteoarthrosis, hand)

Case 11-8
Professional Service: 27355-RT (Excision, Cyst, Femur)

ICD-10-CM: D16.21 (Neoplasm, bone, femur, right side, Benign)

ICD-9-CM: 213.7 (Neoplasm, bone, femur, Benign)

Case 11-9
Professional Service: 29848-LT (Arthroscopy, Surgical, Wrist)

ICD-10-CM: G56.02 (Syndrome, carpal tunnel)

ICD-9-CM: 354.0 (Carpal tunnel syndrome)

Case 11-10
Professional Service: 29877-LT (Arthroscopy, Surgical, Knee)

ICD-10-CM: M94.262 (Chondromalacia, knee), **M22.42** (Chondromalacia, patella)

ICD-9-CM: 733.92 (Chondromalacia, tibial plateau), **717.7** (Chondromalacia, knee/patella)

Case 11-11
Professional Service: 27327-LT (Excision, Tumor, Knee)

ICD-10-CM: D21.22 (Neoplasm, connective tissue, knee, Benign)

ICD-9-CM: 215.3 (Neoplasm, connective tissue, knee, Benign)

Case 11-12
Professional Service: 26160-F7 (Excision, Cyst, Finger), **26055-51-F7** (Incision, Finger, Tendon Sheath)

ICD-10-CM: M67.441 (Ganglion [tendon sheath], hand)

ICD-9-CM: 727.42 (Cyst, tendon sheath)

Case 11-13
Professional Service: 27130-RT (Arthroplasty, Hip, Total Replacement)

ICD-10-CM: M16.11 (Osteoarthritis, hip)

ICD-9-CM: 715.95 (Osteoarthrosis, pelvic region or thigh)

CHAPTER 12: OTORHINOLARYNGOLOGY

Case 12-1
Professional Service: 69436-RT (Tympanostomy)

ICD-10-CM: T85.698A (Complication, prosthetic device or implant, specified, mechanical, obstruction), **H65.491** (Otitis, media, nonsuppurative, chronic), **H61.21** (Impaction, impacted, cerumen [ear] [external])

ICD-9-CM: 996.59 (Complication, mechanical, implant NEC), **381.3** (Otitis, media, chronic with effusion), **380.4** (Wax in ear)

Case 12-2
Professional Service: 31541 (Laryngoscopy, Direct)

ICD-10-CM: C32.0 (Neoplasm, vocal cords [true], Malignant Primary), **R49.0** (Hoarseness)

ICD-9-CM: 161.0 (Neoplasm, vocal cords, true, Malignant, Primary), **784.42** (Hoarseness)

Case 12-3
Professional Service: 69436-LT (Tympanostomy), **69424-59-RT** (Ventilating Tube, Removal)

ICD-10-CM: H66.91 (Otitis, media), **T85.628A** (Complication, prosthetic device or implant, specified NEC, mechanical, displacement), **H65.492** (Otitis media, nonsuppurative, chronic), **H66.91** (Otitis, media), **H72.91** (Perforation, tympanic membrane)

ICD-9-CM: 996.59 (Complication, mechanical, device NEC), **381.3** (Otitis media, chronic, with effusion), **382.9** (Otitis, media), **384.20** (Perforation/perforative, tympanum)

Case 12-4
Professional Service: 42830 (Adenoids, Excision), **30930-51** (Fracture, Nasal Turbinates, Therapeutic)

ICD-10-CM: J34.3 (Hypertrophy, nasal, turbinate), **J35.2** (Hypertrophy, adenoids [infective])

ICD-9-CM: 478.0 (Hypertrophy, nasal, turbinate), **474.12** (Hypertrophy, adenoids)

Case 12-5
Professional Service: 42820 (Tonsils, Excision, with Adenoids)

ICD-10-CM: J35.01 (Tonsillitis, chronic), **G47.33** (Apnea, sleep, obstructive [adult] [pediatric])

ICD-9-CM: 474.00 (Tonsillitis, chronic), **327.23** (Apnea, sleep, obstructive [adult] [pediatric])

Case 12-6
Professional Service: 43200 (Endoscopy, Esophagus, Exploration), **43450-51** (Dilation, Esophagus)

ICD-10-CM: K22.2 (Stricture, esophagus), **R13.10** (Dysphagia), **K20.9** (Esophagitis)

ICD-9-CM: 530.3 (Stricture, esophagus), **787.20** (Dysphagia), **530.10** (Esophagitis)

Case 12-7
Professional Service: 38510-LT (Biopsy, Lymph Nodes)

ICD-10-CM: C77.0 (Neoplasm, lymph gland, cervical, Malignant, Secondary), **C80.1** (Neoplasm, unknown site, Malignant, Primary)

ICD-9-CM: 196.0 (Neoplasm, lymph gland, cervical, Secondary, Malignant), **199.1** (Neoplasm, unknown site, Primary, Malignant)

Case 12-8
Professional Service: 30520 (Septoplasty), **21320-51** (Fracture, Nasal Bone, Closed Treatment)

ICD-10-CM: S02.2xxA (Fracture, traumatic, nose [bone] [septum]), **J34.2** (Deviation, septum [nasal] [acquired]), **W21.03xA** (External Cause Index, Struck [accidentally] by, sports equipment, ball, baseball), **Y93.64** (External Cause Index, Activity [involving], baseball)

ICD-9-CM: 802.0 (Fracture, nose [bone] [closed]), **470** (Deviation, septum [acquired] [nasal]), **E917.0** (Index to External Causes, Striking against, object, moving, in, sports), **E007.3** (Index to External Causes, Activity, Softball)

Case 12-9
Professional Service: 21462-LT (Fracture, Mandible, Open Treatment, with Interdental Fixation)

ICD-10-CM: S02.65xA (Fracture, traumatic, mandible, angle of jaw), **Y04.0xxA** (External Code Index, Assault, fight)

ICD-9-CM: 802.25 (Fracture, mandible, angle), **E960.0** (Index to External Causes, Fight)

Case 12-10
Professional Service: 42815 (Excision, Cyst, Branchial)

ICD-10-CM: Q18.0 (Cyst, branchial [cleft])

ICD-9-CM: 744.42 (Cyst, branchial [cleft])

Case 12-11
Professional Service: 69650-LT (Mobilization, Stapes)

ICD-10-CM: H90.6 (Deafness, conductive, and sensorineural, mixed, bilateral), **H74.02** (Tympanosclerosis)

ICD-9-CM: 389.22 (Loss, hearing, conductive [air], with sensorineural hearing loss, bilateral), **385.02** (Tympanosclerosis, tympanic membrane, with ossicles)

Case 12-12
Professional Service: 30520 (Septoplasty), **31267-51-50** (Antrostomy, Sinus, Maxillary), **31288-51-50** (Sphenoidotomy, Excision with Nasal/Sinus Endoscopy), **31255-51-50** (Ethmoidectomy, Endoscopic), **30930-51-50** (Turbinate, Fracture, Therapeutic)

ICD-10-CM: J34.2 (Deviation, septum), **J33.9** (Polyp, nasal), **J33.8** (Polyp, sinus), **J32.4** (Pansinusitis), **J34.3** (Hypertrophy, nasal, turbinate)

ICD-9-CM: 470 (Deviation, septum), **471.9** (Polyp, nasal), **471.8** (Polyp, sinus [accessory]), **473.8** (Pansinusitis), **478.0** (Hypertrophy, turbinate)

Case 12-13
Professional Service: 67880-LT (Suture, Eyelid)

ICD-10-CM: H02.106 (Ectropion, eyelid [paralytic], left, unspecified lid)

ICD-9-CM: 374.12 (Ectropion, eyelid, paralytic)

CHAPTER 13: PATHOLOGY

Case 13-1
Professional Service: 88304 (Pathology, Surgical, Gross and Micro Exam, Level III)

ICD-10-CM: M51.26 (Displacement, intervertebral disc, lumbar region)

ICD-9-CM: 722.10 (Displacement, intervertebral disc, lumbar)

Case 13-2
Professional Service: 88307 (Pathology, Surgical, Gross and Micro Exam, Level V)

ICD-10-CM: N80.0 (Adenomyosis), **N83.0** (Cyst, follicular [ovarian]), **D25.1** (Leiomyoma, uterus, intramural), **N87.9** (Dysplasia, cervix)

ICD-9-CM: 617.0 (Adenomyosis), **620.0** (Cyst, follicular), **218.1** (Leiomyoma, intramural)

Case 13-3
Professional Service: 88307 (Pathology, Surgical, Gross and Micro Exam, Level V)

ICD-10-CM: O41.1430 (Placentitis)

ICD-9-CM: 658.41 (Placentitis, complicating pregnancy)

Case 13-4
Professional Service: 88304 (Pathology, Surgical, Gross and Micro Exam, Level III)

ICD-10-CM: M48.02 (Stenosis, spinal, cervical region)

ICD-9-CM: 723.0 (Stenosis, spinal, cervical)

Case 13-5
Professional Service: 88304 (Pathology, Surgical, Gross and Micro Exam, Level III)

ICD-10-CM: M50.22 (Displacement, intervertebral disc, cervical, cervicothoracic)

ICD-9-CM: 722.0 (Displacement, intervertebral disc, cervical)

Case 13-6
Professional Service: 88305 (Pathology, Surgical, Gross and Micro Exam, Level IV)

ICD-10-CM: N93.8 (Bleeding, uterus, dysfunctional of functional)

ICD-9-CM: 626.8 (Bleeding, uterus, dysfunctional)

Case 13-7
Professional Service: 88304 (Pathology, Surgical, Gross and Micro Exam, Level III)

ICD-10-CM: I61.9 (Hemorrhage, intracranial, intracerebral [nontraumatic])

ICD-9-CM: 431 (Hematoma, brain, nontraumatic)

Case 13-8
Professional Service: 88304 (Pathology, Surgical, Gross and Micro Exam, Level III)

ICD-10-CM: L02.224 (Furuncle, groin), **E11.9** (Diabetes, diabetic)

ICD-9-CM: 680.2 (Boil, groin), **250.00** (Diabetes, diabetic)

Case 13-9
Professional Service: 88305 (Pathology, Surgical, Gross and Micro Exam, Level IV) Note: Do not report 88331 as it would be reported with the frozen section.

ICD-10-CM: D15.1 (Neoplasm, heart, Benign)

ICD-9-CM: 212.7 (Neoplasm, heart, Benign)

Case 13-10
Professional Service: 88305 (Pathology, Surgical Gross and Micro Exam, Level IV)

ICD-10-CM: M60.9 (Myositis)

ICD-9-CM: 728.9 (Inflammation, muscle)

CHAPTER 14: PEDIATRICS, NEONATOLOGY, AND ADOLESCENT MEDICINE

Case 14-1
Professional Service: 99391 (Preventive Medicine, Established Patient)

ICD-10-CM: Z00.129 (Examination, child [over 28 days old])

ICD-9-CM: V20.32 (Checkup, newborn, routine, subsequent)

Case 14-2
Professional Service: 99468 (Neonatal Critical Care, Initial)

ICD-10-CM: P07.17 (Low birth weight, 1750-1999 grams), **P07.31** (Preterm infant, newborn, with gestation of, 28-31 weeks), **P22.0** (Hyaline, membrane), **P71.8** (Hypermagnesemia, neonatal), **Z84.81** (History, family [of], genetic disease carrier)

ICD-9-CM: 765.17 (Preterm infant), **765.26** (Newborn, gestation, 31–32 completed weeks), **769** (Hyaline, membrane), **775.5** (Hypermagnesemia, neonatal), **V18.9** (History, family, carrier, genetic disease)

Case 14-3
Professional Service: 99469 (Critical Care Services, Neonatal, Subsequent)

ICD-10-CM: P07.17 (Low birth weight, 1750-1999 grams), **P07.31** (Preterm infant, newborn, gestation, 28-31 weeks), **P22.0** (Hyaline, membrane), **P74.4** (Imbalance, electrolyte, neonatal, transitory NEC), **P59.9** (Jaundice, newborn)

ICD-9-CM: 765.17 (Preterm newborn), **765.25** (Newborn, gestation, 29–30 completed weeks), **769** (Hyaline, membrane [disease] [lung] [newborn]), **775.5** (Imbalance, electrolyte, neonatal), **774.6** (Hyperbilirubinemia, neonatal)

Case 14-4
Professional Service: 99469 (Critical Care Services, Neonatal, Subsequent)

ICD-10-CM: P07.17 (Low birth weight, 1750-1999 grams), **P07.31** (Preterm infant, newborn, with gestation of, 28-31 weeks), **P22.0** (Hyaline, membrane), **P59.9** (Jaundice, newborn), **Q25.0** (Patent ductus arteriosus or Botallo)

ICD-9-CM: 765.17 (Pre-term, infant), **765.25** (Newborn, gestation, 29–30 completed weeks), **769** (Hyaline, membrane), **774.6** (Hyperbilirubinemia, neonatal), **747.0** (Patent ductus arteriosus or Botallo)

Case 14-5
Professional Service: 54150 (Circumcision, Surgical, Newborn)

ICD-10-CM: N47.1 (Phimosis)

ICD-9-CM: 605 (Phimosis)

Case 14-6
Professional Service: 10/1: **99460**, 10/2: **99462**, 10/3: **99462-25**, 10/4: **99462** (Evaluation and Management, Newborn Care), 10/3: **54150** (Circumcision, Surgical, Newborn), 10/5: **99238-24** (Evaluation and Management, Hospital, Discharge)

ICD-10-CM: Z38.00 (Newborn [infant] [liveborn] [single], born in hospital)

ICD-9-CM: V30.00 (Newborn, single, born in hospital [without mention of cesarean delivery or section])

CHAPTER 15: DIAGNOSTIC RADIOLOGY

Case 15-1
Professional Service: 70450-26 (CT Scan, without Contrast, Head)

ICD-10-CM: I60.9 (Hemorrhage, intracranial [nontraumatic], subarachnoid [nontraumatic] [from])

ICD-9-CM: 430 (Hemorrhage, subarachnoid [nontraumatic])

Case 15-2
Professional Service: 71020-26 (X-Ray, Chest)

ICD-10-CM: J90 (Effusion, pleura)

ICD-9-CM: 511.9 (Effusion, pleura)

Case 15-3
Professional Service: 70450-26 (CT Scan, without Contrast, Head)

ICD-10-CM: R41.82 (Alteration [of], Altered, mental status)

ICD-9-CM: 780.97 (Alteration, mental status)

Case 15-4
Professional Service: 71020-26 (X-Ray, Chest)

ICD-10-CM: J18.9 (Pneumonia)

ICD-9-CM: 486 (Pneumonia)

Case 15-5
Professional Service: 74176-26 (CT Scan, without Contrast, Abdomen)

ICD-10-CM: R18.8 (Ascites)

ICD-9-CM: 789.59 (Ascites)

Case 15-6
Professional Service: 76705-26 (Ultrasound, Abdomen)

ICD-10-CM: E80.6 (Disorder, bilirubin excretion)

ICD-9-CM: 277.4 (Findings, abnormal, bilirubin)

Case 15-7
Professional Service: 76770-26 (Ultrasound, Retroperitoneal)

ICD-10-CM: R94.4 (Findings/abnormal/inconclusive, without diagnosis, function study, kidney)

ICD-9-CM: 794.4 (Findings, abnormal, without diagnosis, function study, kidney)

Case 15-8
Professional Service: 36558 (Insertion, Catheter, Venous Access Device), **77001-26** (Fluoroscopy, Venous Access Device)

ICD-10-CM: N18.6 (Disease, renal, end-stage [failure])

ICD-9-CM: 585.6 (Disease, end-stage, renal)

Case 15-9
Professional Service: 78452-26 (Stress Tests, Myocardial Perfusion Imaging)

ICD-10-CM: R07.9 (Pain, chest), **I25.10** (Disease, heart, ischemic, atherosclerotic), **Z95.2** (Status, organ replacement, by artificial or mechanical device or prosthesis of, heart, valve)

ICD-9-CM: 786.50 (Pain, chest), **410.01** (Arteriosclerosis, coronary [artery], native artery), **V43.3** (Status, organ replacement, heart, valve)

Case 15-10
Professional Service: 78582-26 (Lung, Nuclear Medicine, Imaging, Perfusion)

ICD-10-CM: J81.1 (Edema, lung)

ICD-9-CM: 514 (Edema, lung)

Case 15-11
Professional Service: 76506-26 (Echoencephalography)

ICD-10-CM: P07.17 (Low birthweight, 1750-1999 grams), **P07.30** (Preterm infant, newborn)

ICD-9-CM: 765.17 (Preterm infant), **765.20** (Newborn, gestation, unspecified completed weeks)

Case 15-12
Professional Service: 74000-26 (Abdomen, X-Ray)

ICD-10-CM: Z45.2 (Admission [for], adjustment [of], device, vascular access)

ICD-9-CM: V58.81 (Admission for, adjustment of, catheter, vascular)

Case 15-13
Professional Service: 74455-26 (Urethrocystography)

ICD-10-CM: Q62.0 (Hydronephrosis, congenital)

ICD-9-CM: 753.29 (Hydronephrosis, congenital)

CHAPTER 16: INTERVENTIONAL RADIOLOGY AND RADIATION ONCOLOGY

Case 16-1
Professional Service: 47000 (Biopsy, Liver), **77012-26** (CT Scan, Guidance, Needle Placement)

ICD-10-CM: C22.8 (Neoplasm, liver, Malignant Primary)

ICD-9-CM: 155.0 (Neoplasm, liver, Malignant, Primary)

Case 16-2
Professional Service: 32405-RT (Biopsy, Lung, Needle), **77012-26** (CT Scan, Guidance, Needle Placement)

ICD-10-CM: C34.31 (Neoplasm, lung, lower lobe, Malignant Primary)

ICD-9-CM: 162.5 (Neoplasm, lung, lower lobe, Malignant, Primary)

Case 16-3
Professional Service: 62270 (Puncture, Spinal Cord, Diagnostic), **76000-26** (Fluoroscopy, Hourly)

ICD-10-CM: R51 (Headache)

ICD-9-CM: 784.0 (Headache)

Case 16-4
Professional Service: 49083 (Abdomen, Drainage, Fluid), **99144** (Sedation, Moderate)

ICD-10-CM: R18.8 (Ascites, abdominal), **K74.60** (Cirrhosis)

ICD-9-CM: 789.59 (Ascites, abdominal), **571.5** (Cirrhosis)

Case 16-5
Professional Service: 36558 (Insertion, Catheter, Venous), **77001-26** (Fluoroscopy, Venous Access Device), **99144, 99145** (Sedation, Moderate)

ICD-10-CM: C34.90 (Neoplasm, lung, lobe NEC, Malignant Primary)

ICD-9-CM: 162.9 (Neoplasm, lung, Malignant, Primary)

Case 16-6
Professional Service: 36217-RT (Catheterization, Brachiocephalic Artery), **36218-RT** (Catheterization, Thoracic), **75650-26** (Angiography, Head, Artery), **75671-26** (Angiography, Carotid Artery), **75680-26** (Angiography, Carotid Artery, Cervical, Bilateral)

ICD-10-CM: I65.22 (Occlusion, artery, carotid)

ICD-9-CM: 433.10 (Narrowing, artery, carotid)

Case 16-7
Professional Service: 36217-RT (Catheterization, Thoracic Artery), **36218-RT** (Catheterization, Thoracic Artery), **36215-59-51-LT** (Catheterization, Thoracic Artery), **75650-26** (Angiography, Head, Artery), **75671-26** (Angiography, Carotid Artery), **75680-26** (Angiography, Carotid Artery, Cervical, Bilateral), **75685-26** (Angiography, Vertebral)

ICD-10-CM: I65.23 (Occlusion, artery, carotid)

ICD-9-CM: 433.30 (Occlusion, artery, carotid, with other precerebral artery, bilateral)

Case 16-8
Professional Service: 49452-52 (Replacement, Gastrostomy Tube)

ICD-10-CM: K94.23 (Complication, gastrostomy, mechanical)

ICD-9-CM: 536.42 (Complication, mechanical, gastrostomy)

Case 16-9
Professional Service: 36147 (Catheterization, Arterio-venous Shunt), **75791-26** (Angiography, Arteriovenous Shunt)

ICD-10-CM: T82.898A (Complication, arteriovenous, fistula, surgically created, specified type NEC), **I86.8** (Varix, specified site, NEC), **N18.6** (Failure, renal, end-stage), **Z99.2** (Dialysis, renal, status)

ICD-9-CM: 996.73 (Complication, due to [presence of] any device, implant or graft classified), **456.8** (Aneurysm, venous), **586** (Failure, renal, end stage), **V45.11** (Status, dialysis)

Case 16-10
Professional Service: 36247-RT (Catheterization, Legs), **37201** (Transcatheter Therapy, Infusion), **75896-26** (Transcatheter Therapy, Infusion), **75710-59-26-RT** (Angiography, Leg Artery)

ICD-10-CM: T82.392A (Complication, extremity artery [bypass] graft, mechanical, obstruction, femoral artery), **I74.3** (Thrombosis, thrombotic, leg, arterial)

ICD-9-CM: 996.74 (Complication, due to (presence of) any device, implant or graft, arterial), **440.22** (Thrombosis, thrombotic, femoral)

Case 16-11
Professional Service: 36246-LT (Catheterization, Legs), **75625-26** (Aortography, Serial), **75716-26** (Angiography, Leg Artery)

ICD-10-CM: I70.244 (Arteriosclerosis, extremities, leg, left with, ulceration [and intermittent claudication and rest pain], heel), **I70.201** (Arteriosclerosis, extremities, leg, right), **I70.92** (Occlusion, artery, total [chronic], extremities), **L97.429** (Ulcer, lower limb, heel, left), **Z94.0** (Transplant, kidney)

ICD-9-CM: 440.23 (Arteriosclerosis, extremities, ulceration), **440.4** (Occlusion, extremities, complete), **707.14** (Ulcer, heel), **V42.0** (Transplant, kidney)

Case 16-12
Professional Service: 99255 (Evaluation and Management, Consultation)

ICD-10-CM: C34.90 (Neoplasm, lung, unspecified site, unspecified side, Malignant Primary), **Z99.1** (Dependence on ventilator)

ICD-9-CM: 162.9 (Neoplasm, lung, Primary, Malignant), **V46.11** (Status, ventilator [respirator])

Case 16-13
Professional Service: 77261 (Radiation Therapy, Planning)

ICD-10-CM: C34.90 (Neoplasm, lung, lobe NEC, Malignant Primary)

ICD-9-CM: 162.9 (Neoplasm, lung, Malignant, Primary)

Case 16-14
Professional Service: 77280 (Radiation Therapy, Field Set-Up)

ICD-10-CM: C34.90 (Neoplasm, lung, lobe NEC, Malignant Primary)

ICD-9-CM: 162.9 (Neoplasm, lung, Malignant, Primary)

CHAPTER 17: UROLOGY

Case 17-1
Professional Service: 50200-LT (Biopsy, Kidney)

ICD-10-CM: R31.9 (Hematuria, unspecified)

ICD-9-CM: 599.70 (Hematuria)

Case 17-2
Professional Service: 52000 (Cystoscopy)

ICD-10-CM: C67.2 (Neoplasm, bladder, wall, lateral, Malignant, Primary)

ICD-9-CM: 188.2 (Neoplasm, bladder, wall, lateral, Primary, Malignant)

Case 17-3
Professional Service: 51702 (Insertion, Catheter, Bladder)

ICD-10-CM: T83.89xA (Complication, catheter, urethral, indwelling)

ICD-9-CM: 996.76 (Complications, urethral catheter)

Case 17-4
Professional Service: 52005 (Cystourethroscopy, Catheterization, Ureteral), **74420-26** (Urography, Retrograde)

ICD-10-CM: N40.0 (Enlargement, prostate, without urinary retention [LUTS])

ICD-9-CM: 600.90 (Hyperplasia, prostate)

Case 17-5
Professional Service: 50200-RT (Biopsy, Kidney), **76942-26** (Ultrasound, Guidance, Needle Biopsy)

ICD-10-CM: R31.0 (Hematuria, gross), **N17.9** (Failure, renal, acute)

ICD-9-CM: 599.71 (Hematuria, gross), **584.9** (Failure, renal, acute)

Case 17-6
Professional Service: 50200-LT (Biopsy, Kidney)

ICD-10-CM: N04.9 (Syndrome, nephrotic)

ICD-9-CM: 581.9 (Syndrome, nephrotic)

Case 17-7
Professional Service: 52332-RT (Cystourethroscopy, Insertion, Indwelling Ureteral Stent)

ICD-10-CM: Z46.6 (Admission for, removal of, ureteral stent), **N13.5** (Stricture, ureter [postoperative]), **N30.40** (Cystitis, irradiation), **Y84.2** (External Cause Index, Complication of or following radiologic procedure or therapy), **Z85.42** (History, personal, malignant neoplasm [of], uterus)

ICD-9-CM: V53.6 (Admission for, removal of, ureteral stent), **593.3** (Stricture, ureter), **595.82** (Cystitis, irradiation), **E879.2** (Index to External Causes, Radiation, abnormal reaction to medical test or therapy), **V10.42** (History, personal, malignant neoplasm, uterus)

Case 17-8
Professional Service: 52240 (Cystourethroscopy, with Fulguration, Tumor)

ICD-10-CM: C67.2 (Neoplasm, bladder, wall, lateral, Malignant, Primary)

ICD-9-CM: 188.9 (Neoplasm, bladder, Malignant, Primary)

Case 17-9
Professional Service: 52005 (Cystourethroscopy, with Ureteral Catheterization), **54161-51** (Circumcision, Surgical Excision), **54060** (Penis, Lesion, Surgical Excision), **74420-26** (Urography, Retrograde)

ICD-10-CM: N20.0 (Calculus, kidney), **A63.0** (Condyloma, acuminatum)

ICD-9-CM: 592.0 (Calculus, renal), **078.11** (Condyloma, acuminatum)

Case 17-10
Professional Service: 54324 (Hypospadias, Repair, Urethroplasty, Local Skin Flaps), **55060-51-RT**, (Hydrocele, Repair)

ICD-10-CM: Q54.1 (Hypospadias, penile), **Q54.4** (Chordee, congenital), **N43.3** (Hydrocele)

ICD-9-CM: 752.61 (Hypospadias, male), **752.63** (Chordee, congenital), **603.9** (Hydrocele)

CHAPTER 18: GENERAL SURGERY

Case 18-1
Professional Service: 44960 (Excision, Appendix)

ICD-10-CM: K35.2 (Appendicitis, with, perforation or rupture)

ICD-9-CM: 540.0 (Appendicitis, with, perforation)

Case 18-2
Professional Service: 49505-RT (Repair, Hernia, Reducible, Inguinal)

ICD-10-CM: K40.90 (Hernia, inguinal, unilateral)

ICD-9-CM: 550.90 (Hernia, inguinal, unilateral)

Case 18-3
Professional Service: 47562 (Cholecystectomy)

ICD-10-CM: K80.20 (Calculus, gallbladder)

ICD-9-CM: 574.20 (Cholelithiasis)

Case 18-4
Professional Service: 20102 (Wound, Exploration, Penetrating, Abdomen/Flank/Back)

ICD-10-CM: S31.140A (Puncture, abdominal, wall, right upper quadrant, with foreign body), **X99.1xxA** (Assault, cutting or piercing instrument, knife)

ICD-9-CM: 879.3 (Wound, open, abdominal, complicated), **E966** (Assault, wound, knife)

Case 18-5
Professional Service: 19120-LT (Excision, Breast Lesion)

ICD-10-CM: D24.02 (Neoplasm, breast, female, unspecified site, Benign)

ICD-9-CM: 217 (Neoplasm, breast, Benign)

Case 18-6
Professional Service: 27590-LT (Amputation, Leg, Upper)

ICD-10-CM: I96 (Gangrene)

ICD-9-CM: 785.4 (Gangrene)

Case 18-7
Professional Service: 49585 (Repair, Hernia, Umbilical)

ICD-10-CM: K42.9 (Hernia, umbilicus, umbilical)

ICD-9-CM: 553.1 (Hernia, umbilical)

Case 18-8
Professional Service: 44626 (Cholecystectomy), **47600-51** (Enterostomy, Closure)

ICD-10-CM: K80.20 (Calculus, gallbladder), **Z43.3** (Admission for, attention to artificial opening, colostomy)

ICD-9-CM: 574.20 (Cholelithiasis), **V55.3** (Admission for, attention to artificial opening, colostomy)

Case 18-9
Professional Service: 19307-RT (Mastectomy, Modified Radical)

ICD-10-CM: C50.911 (Neoplasm, breast, female, unspecified site, Malignant, Primary)

ICD-9-CM: 174.9 (Neoplasm, breast, Malignant, Primary)

Case 18-10
Professional Service: 46040 (Incision and Drainage, Abscess, Rectum)

ICD-10-CM: K61.1 (Abscess, perirectal)

ICD-9-CM: 566 (Abscess, perirectal)

Case 18-11
Professional Service: 49421 (Insertion, Catheter, Abdomen)

ICD-10-CM: N18.6 (Disease, renal, end-stage)

ICD-9-CM: 585.6 (Disease, renal, end stage)

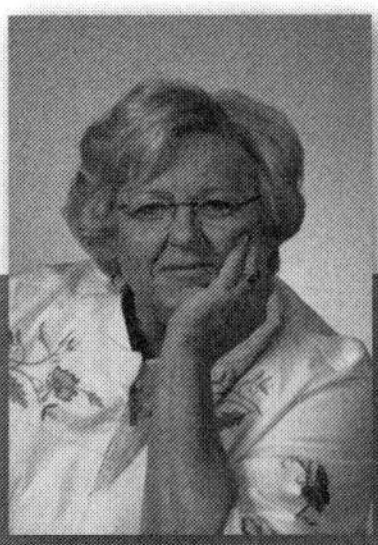